HOLY HEALTH

How Church Makes You Healthier and Happier

PATRICK CHISHOLM

Published by Accentance
PO Box 220402
Chantilly, VA 20153

Cover photos: Runner by Brian A. Jackson via istock.com/Getty Images. Church by Eloyearana via Dreamstime.com (Schönenberg Church/Pilgrimage Church of Our Lady, Ellwangen, Germany).
Illustration and other photo credits: Freepik, Getty Images, Pixabay.
Cover designed with Affinity Photo; interior layout: Adobe InDesign.

ISBNs:
978-1-7376101-1-3 (hc.)
978-1-7376101-0-6 (pbk.)
978-1-7376101-2-0 (ebk.)
978-1-7376101-3-7 (aud.)

Library of Congress control number: 2021914683

First Edition

Every effort has been made to ensure that the information in this book is true and accurate. However it is not intended as a substitute for professional counseling or medical treatment. Significant medical or health-related actions should be done in consultation with a physician. Neither the author nor publisher shall be subject to or responsible for any damage or loss allegedly pertaining to any advice or information within this book.

To Cathy, Aaron, and Ethan

Contents

List of Charts

Personal Stories

Personal Stories, continued...

INTRODUCTION

A t first glance it could be easy to think atheists and agnostics live longer than churchgoers. With no belief in heaven, you might as well strive to achieve health, wealth, and happiness on earth. Why sit in church for an hour Sunday morning when you could spend that time working out at the gym, advancing your career, communing with nature, or sleeping in? Likewise, you'd think churchgoers wouldn't be as concerned as nonbelievers about prolonging their lives, like eating right and keeping fit. After all, a longer earthly life means a longer wait to enter the kingdom of God. But the reality is, churchgoers live longer than non-churchgoers; *six to seven years longer*, on average.[1]

Hand-in-hand with longevity is better overall health. Religion reduces the likelihood of a range of ailments including cancer, heart disease, diabetes, arthritis, asthma, emphysema, tuberculosis, allergies, and diseases of the liver, kidney, and digestive system.[2] Neglecting church is a risk factor in dying an earlier death every bit as much as smoking, heavy drinking, obesity, and inactivity are risk factors.

In addition to better physical health, churchgoers on the whole have better mental health and better life outcomes. As pointed out throughout this book, they're less likely to divorce, get depression, or commit suicide. They're less prone to alcohol and drug abuse, and to unethical or criminal behavior. They have higher educational attainment and higher lifetime earnings. Their kids are more likely to be well adjusted and get better grades.

Religion's positive effect on physical and mental health is the conclusion of literally thousands of peer-reviewed academic studies published in prestigious scholarly journals that have no affiliation with religious institutions whatsoever. They include *JAMA* (Journal of the American Medical Association), *The BMJ* (British Medical Journal), *New England Journal of Medicine, The Lancet, American Journal of Epidemiology, Social Science Research, Journal of Health Psychology, American Sociological Review, American Journal of Psychiatry, Psychological Bulletin, Journal of Personality and Clinical Studies, Preventive Medicine, Demography*, and many more. The investigators are psychologists, sociologists, physicians, epidemiologists, biomedical scientists, nurses, statisticians, economists, and other researchers at hundreds of prominent universities and hospitals. Many if not most of them are agnostics or atheists with no religious axe to grind.

As mentioned in chapter 15, religion is such a compelling factor in health care that even nonreligious psychotherapists and physicians recommend faith-based therapy to their patients. Many nonbelieving scientists choose to go to church, mainly for their kids' benefit (see chapter 8). Some atheists extol religion (chapter 16). Even the prominent militant atheist Richard Dawkins has softened his stance and acknowledged its benefits (chapter 5). Though he didn't choose religion for himself, the French philosopher Voltaire wanted it to be practiced widely in order to reduce crime and vice.

Imagine two sets of people. Both are alike in terms of age, income, and other socioeconomic and demographic characteristics. The only difference is one set of individuals believe in God and regularly attend religious services. Those in the other group have little or no faith and rarely or never attend. "Other things being equal," posited John J. DiIulio, "which group, the first or the second do you suppose suffers less, on average, from hypertension, depression, and drug and alcohol abuse, has lower rates of suicide, non-marital child-bearing, and delinquency, and boasts more members who live into their seventies and eighties?"[3]

The clear answer is the churchgoing group. DiIulio teaches at the University of Pennsylvania and is the former director of the White House Office of Faith-Based and Community Initiatives. He wrote the foreword for a report by Byron R. Johnson (along with

Ralph Brett Tompkins and Derek Webb of UPenn) titled *Objective Hope: Assessing the Effectiveness of Faith-Based Organizations*, which reviewed nearly 800 studies on religiosity's effect on health and wellness, mortality, substance abuse, crime, and other outcomes. In addition to greater "well-being, hope, purpose, meaning in life, and educational attainment," Johnson's review of the literature points to "overwhelming evidence" that religious practices "make for an important protective factor that buffers or insulates individuals from deleterious outcomes."[4] Separately, economist Jonathan Gruber of the Massachusetts Institute of Technology conducted a study concluding that living in an area where there's a larger density of co-religionists prompts people to attend church to a greater extent. That, in turn, leads to all sorts of personal benefits. "My results are striking," he writes. "I find that a higher (religious) market density leads to a significantly increased level of religious participation, and as well to better outcomes according to several key economic indicators: higher levels of education and income, lower levels of welfare receipt and disability, higher levels of marriage, and lower levels of divorce. These results are robust to a variety of specification checks."[5]

Reason for (Well) Being

Religion is normally associated with improving your prospects in the afterlife. Why would it result in so many worldly benefits as well? Among the reasons are that churchgoers often view their lives and physical bodies as gifts from God, motivating them to take better care of themselves. They're less likely to drink and smoke, and are more likely to eat right, follow safety measures such as wear seatbelts, and see the doctor. Some religions or religious denominations prohibit drinking alcohol. That along with less consumption of cigarettes and recreational drugs have obvious long-term benefits. Churchgoers also tend to have more self-discipline, have a greater sense of meaning and purpose, deal with stress better, and tend to steer clear of immoral or unethical activities that could spell trouble later on.

Another standout are the social aspects of organized religion. Churchgoers generally have larger networks of friends, participate in more social activities, and have lower levels of social isolation. The harmful mental and physical effects of loneliness and social isolation are well established, as the psychological fallout from pandemic-related lockdowns attests. As discussed in chapter 2, such circumstances raise stress hormones and inflammation, which in turn boost the risk of heart disease along with cancer, diabetes, dementia, and arthritis.

Social interaction is in our genes; it makes us happier and healthier. For the vast majority of our existence we humans lived in small groups of hunter-gatherers, and later agriculturalists, in which we not only constantly were in the presence of fellow group members but depended on them for survival. We still need that fellowship. Worshiping as a group on a weekly basis or more, along with the many and varied church-related activities, create manifold opportunities to be together and work together. Religious institutions also connect people who share common ideals, purposes, and goals. These aspects help satisfy not only the longing for social interaction but also the desire to be part of something larger than one's self.

Pandemic-related lockdowns attest to the contrasts. Each year the Gallup organization conducts its November Health and Healthcare survey in which Americans rate their mental health. In 2020 in the midst of Covid-19, those deeming their mental health as "excellent" was down substantially from the previous year. This held true for nearly every demographic—male, female, low-income, high-income, old, young, married, nonmarried, Democrat, or Republican—except one demographic: weekly churchgoers. Their numbers actually went up 4 percentage points, with 46 percent of them reporting excellent mental health. It also underscores how important it is to attend church at least once a week. Those attending less than weekly suffered a whopping 12 percentage-point drop, with only 35 percent reporting excellent mental health. For non-churchgoers the plunge was 13 percentage points, to 29 percent.[6]

Religion fosters virtues that improve individuals' lives and society overall. One such virtue is delayed gratification. Churchgoing adults and children are more inclined to practice this than their non-churchgoing counterparts. As disclosed in chapter 5, contemplation of the afterlife no doubt has much to do with it. Those who believe in heaven and hell, and who wish to go to the former and avoid the latter, are prone to avoid activities they would find gratifying yet consider to be sinful, whether it be excessive drinking, overeating, illegal drugs, unchastity, envy, anger, and a host of other vices. For kids it could mean doing their homework instead of spending hours playing video games. The perception that a higher being or beings are watching your every move, and that punishment awaits misbehavers in the afterlife, can make a model citizen out of even the most pitiful would-be scoundrel.

Perhaps the biggest reason for life satisfaction among churchgoers are the direct benefits received from God, known as graces. Separate from the thousands of conventional studies on the religion-health relationship, there's a small genre of studies that seek to test the effectiveness of prayer. As highlighted in chapter 13, most of them show that prayer really works. Given the existence of a loving God, humbly petitioning Him is bound to bear fruit. There also are numerous accounts of miraculous healings from prayer. But this book isn't about that. For the vast majority of churchgoers, better wellness comes from various subtle influences, behaviors, attitudes, and modes of thinking. It's those small graces that have a significant cumulative effect.

And it's active worship that counts. Considering yourself religious but routinely skipping church or synagogue isn't likely to yield the same benefits. It even could be somewhat worse; Israeli Jews of lukewarm religiosity were shown to have inferior physical and mental health than secular Jews.[7]

Holy is Holistic

In a variety of aspects of life, religion and particularly churchgoing brings with it a range of benefits. Holy health is the pathway to holistic health. It's physical, emotional, social, and spiritual wellness. Based on numerous peer-reviewed scientific studies, following is a partial list of the (earthly) benefits churchgoers are more likely to enjoy:[8]

Physical Health
Longer lifespan
Improved cardiovascular function
Lower risk of stroke
Less coronary artery disease
Less cancer
Improved immune system
Better endocrine function
Fewer diseases of various kinds
Faster recovery rates
More frequent doctor and dentist visits
More exercise/physical activity
Healthier diet
Lower disability among elderly
Slower progression of Alzheimer's disease
Fewer sexually transmitted diseases

Mental and Emotional Health
Less depression
Less anxiety
Less suicide and suicide ideation
Fewer eating disorders
Lower stress levels
Greater sense of well-being
Greater happiness
Greater sense of hope and optimism
Greater sense of meaning and purpose
Larger social networks
Better coping skills
Greater self-control/self-discipline
Greater self-esteem
Greater ability to forgive

Marriage and Family
Stronger marriages
Less divorce
Greater marital happiness
More satisfying marriages
More satisfying marital sexual intimacy
More stable families
Better-behaved children
Better parent-child relationships
Lower rates of teen sex
Fewer out-of-wedlock births
Lower cohabitation rates

Education and Productivity
Greater self-discipline
Better grades in school
Higher educational attainment
Greater work productivity
Better work habits
Better cooperation

Charity
Higher levels of charitable donations
Greater volunteerism
Greater helpfulness and good-neighborliness

Law Abidance
Less criminal behavior
Lower rates of juvenile crime and delinquency
Lower violent crime
Lower recidivism
Less domestic abuse and violence

Substance Abuse and Other
Less alcohol consumption
Less binge drinking
Less illegal drug use
Less prescription drug misuse
Less marijuana use

Faster recovery from drug or alcohol addiction
Less cigarette smoking and vaping
Less pathological gambling
Less porn addiction

Ironies Abound

Note the ironies here. We live in a culture where health-conscious-ness is all the rage. People pay more for all-natural and organic foods. They eat whole grains. They drink plenty of water. They avoid saturated fats, excess sodium, and high-fructose corn syrup. They make sure to get enough omega-3 fatty acids. They swallow vitamins and nutrition supplements. They wear their Fitbits and step-counters. They're religious about going to the gym. There are weight-loss programs galore. Restaurants put calorie counts and fat content on their menus. There's a focus on "healthy aging." On the mental health side, in addition to taking antidepressants they practice mindfulness meditation, yoga, relaxation techniques, deep-breathing exercises, and pet therapy. They heed advice to get enough sleep, smile more, laugh more, get "off the grid," and take nature walks. The younger generation is said to be even more health conscious than older generations.

Yet they're closing their eyes to a major health enhancer, despite the thousands of studies attesting to its effectiveness. And it shows. With the revolution in health foods and fitness, you'd think life expectancy in America would be skyrocketing. It isn't. After rising for centuries (apart from the Civil War and Spanish flu years), it peaked at 78.9 years of age in 2014 and then leveled off and even declined somewhat thereafter.[9] The healthy-habits trend no doubt prevented an even greater decline. But on the negative side there's a more powerful trend: "deaths of despair"—from suicide, drug overdoses, and alcohol abuse. The rise of the unchurched is a key driver. As pointed out in chapter 10, nearly 40 percent of the upsurge in the suicide rate in recent decades stems from the drop-off in church attendance.[10] That same drop-off is helping to fuel drug and alcohol deaths. Suicides and mental illness are highest in the younger generation, even though they're the most health conscious. Why the disconnect? A big reason is they're the least religious.

Another irony is the institution that's generating all of these studies: academia. Long known for the atheists and agnostics who dominate their lecture halls, colleges and universities neverthe-less are churning out study after study, paper after paper, on the positive association between religiosity and health. These studies aren't coming from small fundamentalist colleges in the middle of Bible Belt, U.S.A. They're coming from the most well-known and prestigious universities in the United States and the world: Harvard, Yale, MIT, Stanford, and hundreds of other big-name universities and colleges not known as bastions of spiritual belief. But in this case, any anti-religious bias seems to be held at bay. While there's still some resistance, professors are largely free to study the prac-tical benefits of religion.[11] Such academic freedom is how it should be; the mission of academia is supposed to be the pursuit of truth, even if that truth goes against prevailing assumptions. After all, the motto of many secular colleges and universities, sometimes etched in stone on main buildings, is, "Ye shall know the truth and the truth shall set you free." The motto is taken from the Bible, uttered by Jesus Christ.

Putting God First

The many benefits listed above are compelling reasons to go to church. But be careful. This isn't the "prosperity Gospel." Diligently worshiping God and generously giving to the poor won't necessar-ily mean God will repay you with financial success, good health, and happiness. He may, but only if He thinks it will help you live a holier life, be closer to Him, be an inspiration to your children or grandchildren, and spread His Word to others. God's overarching desire is for you to spend eternity with Him in heaven, not for you to live it up during your short time here on earth. All too often, material benefits pull people away from God. It's one reason why as countries grow wealthier, they tend to become less religious. The love of money is the root of all evil, writes St. Paul. (1 Timothy

6:10) In addition to money, modern-day false gods include fitness, health foods, sports, the quest for fun, the quest for comfort, and the pursuit of longevity. Not that these are bad; the problem is when a person focuses only on them, while neglecting God. Often the only time people do turn to Him is during bouts of distress or tragedy. God knows whether you're that type of person. If you start taking your faith more seriously and He thinks you need to take it even more seriously, then He may decide against mending your ailing body or healing your broken heart. He may ask you to take up your cross and follow Him. (Luke 9:23)

But if you have the right attitude He may opt to grant you unexpected rewards. That's what happened to King Solomon in the Old Testament. Most kings during that time were after wealth, long life, power, and glory. When asked in a dream what he wanted from God, King Solomon expressed humility and appealed for wisdom and the ability to distinguish right from wrong. God was pleased with that answer, rewarding him with wisdom, riches, longevity, abundant offspring, and peace with surrounding nations. (1 Kings 3:1-15) He was a faithful servant of God for most of his kingship— until toward the end of his life. The pleasures of the world caught up with him, with his hundreds of wives and concubines. To please them he put up temples to false gods. His devotion to the one true God waned. The king's good fortune then took a turn for the worse in the form of new foreign adversaries to worry about. (1 Kings 11:1-25) The lesson: never let your faith grow cold, and never get too attached to worldly pursuits.

In response to the flurry of academic literature on the religion-health connection, scholars have cautioned against embracing church for the secondary reason of improving your wellness rather than the main purpose for which religious institutions were established. Studies linking religion and health can lead people to become religious just for the sake of health, rather than for the sake of God. There's a risk of missing true meaning in favor of a type of self-interested individualism.[12] Religious traditions teach not how to be healthy and live long, but how to live and die faithfully, write

Joel James Shuman and Keith Meador in their book *Heal Thyself: Spirituality, Medicine, and the Distortion of Christianity.* "Prioritizing the immediate benefits of being religious over the requirements of faithfulness, many of those same traditions have a name: idolatry."[13]

As neuroscientist Andrew Newberg of the University of Pennsylvania observed, "You can't pretend to be religious in order to get its health-related effects. You're religious because you believe in it. And if it has health benefits, then that's just an added bonus."[14]

From a Christian perspective, to paraphrase C.S. Lewis, you should be a Christian because you really want to follow the teachings of Jesus Christ and worship him, not because of any worldly benefits that come with being a Christian. The spiritual dividends are the true prize; the goal of eternal life with God is far more important than any physical or emotional benefits here on earth. Going to church solely for temporal rewards is the sin of pride—in which it's done for the love of self rather than the love of God. A second-century sermon, believed to be the earliest complete Christian sermon in written form (outside of the New Testament) and attributed to St. Clement of Rome, contains the admonition, "If God gave the reward of the righteous after a short time, we would immediately be exercising ourselves in business, not in godliness. We would seem to be righteous while pursuing not what is godly, but what is profitable."[15] So it behooves us to not show up at church out of motives of worldly gain.

But what if you're convinced church would be a good thing from a physical and emotional standpoint, but your faith in God is weak or nonexistent? Go there anyway, and stick with it. You may come around to believing—whether it be through getting touched by the Holy Spirit, through being inspired by those around you, through becoming convinced by the compelling evidence of the existence of God and authenticity of the Gospels (see last chapter), or any number of other reasons. Before long, your primary motivation will be love for God—and there's a good chance you'll still reap the worldly benefits to boot. Changes in outlook may call for sacrificing some things you previously enjoyed that drew you away from the

Lord, but new kinds of enjoyments await. "For my yoke is easy, and my burden light." (Matthew 11:30)

Bear in Mind

Throughout this book, keep in mind the following important points:

• "Church," "churchgoing," and Sunday worship are used for simplicity's sake. The health advantages discussed here apply not only to churches but to mosques, synagogues, and temples, whether their holy day is Friday, Saturday, or Sunday. Also, "churchgoing" for purposes of this book refers to regular churchgoing, on a weekly basis or more.

• Most of the studies on the religion-health relationship involve the Christian faith because the vast majority of them were carried out in the United States and other Christian-majority countries. Even so, studies involving non-Christians are highlighted in this book as well.

• Virtually all of the studies cited here control for various factors such as age, gender, income, race/ethnicity, socioeconomic status, geographic region, prior health status, and health-related behaviors. That is, regardless of the extent to which the person is affected by these factors, the favorable effect of religion still holds. Sophisticated statistical methods are used to ensure the factors are separated out so as to not skew the outcome. This also is helpful in ruling out the possibility of reverse causation whereby rather than religion leading to health, those who are already healthy are more predisposed to being religious.

• Frequently cited in this book are longitudinal studies, which involve gathering data over time, usually a period of years. Cross-sectional studies, by contrast, get data from a single point in time. Longitudinal studies typically are considered more reliable.

• In measuring the effects of religiosity on health and longevity, researchers often focus on older persons since they're far more likely to get sick and die than younger adults. In epidemiology (i.e., the study and analysis of factors that affect health in specified populations) the old can make much better research subjects than the young since in longitudinal work it takes a lot less time before ill health effects start showing up. This book mentions several studies done on the elderly. So if you're young or middle-aged, don't get the impression from these studies that health benefits of church and prayer don't apply to you. They certainly do, albeit perhaps in more subtle ways. Besides, you'll be in those older folks' shoes someday yourself.

- Many studies cited here go back to the 1990s and early 2000s, as that was when extensive groundbreaking work in religion and health was carried out. Those studies are still very relevant today. Instead of repeating previous work, more recent studies on this topic often get more specialized—too narrow in scope for the purposes of this book.* But other recent ones are still quite noteworthy, discussed in the pages that follow.

- When the affiliation of authors and investigators is mentioned, it's the affiliation at the time their study was published. Since then, many of them have moved to other institutions and a few have even, God rest their souls, passed away. Also, assume nearly all have "Dr." in front of their name, either M.D.'s or Ph.D.'s.

- After the first or second mentions in this book, frequently cited leaders in this field typically are referred to simply by last name. They include Harold Koenig of Duke, Tyler VanderWeele of Harvard, Jeff Levin of Baylor, Christopher Ellison of UT San Antonio, Linda Powell of Rush University Medical Center, Annette Mahoney of Bowling Green State, and Patrick Fagan of the Marriage and Religion Research Institute.

---

* Examples include a study evaluating how having interreligious parents during childhood impacts an individual's later religiosity. Another investigated the influence of religiosity on how women cope with prenatal diagnoses of fetal abnormalities. Another sought to discern the mental health and quality of life of persons with multiple religious affiliations versus persons with a single religious affiliation as well as those with no religious affiliation. Other recent studies just focus on particular countries.

Finally, what about bias or self-censorship that could inflate the number of studies pointing to a positive association between churchgoing and wellness? In the academic arena there's something known as the "file-drawer effect," in which the results are contrary to the prediction or hypothesis, prompting the quiet shelving of the study without having it published. In the area of religion and health, Yoichi Chida and Andrew Steptoe of University College London along with Rush University's Linda Powell don't think the file-drawer effect is much in play. They analyzed dozens of studies on the subject, pointing out that "the fail-safe number in the overall analysis of healthy population studies was sufficiently high that a very large number of nonsignificant studies would have to be in the 'file drawer' to negate the significance of the association."[16]

Apart from that, given that so many in academia are agnostics or atheists and that increasing numbers are virulently anti-Christian, one would think the less scrupulous among them would be more prone to put into the file drawer findings that portray religion in a positive light. So it speaks volumes that there are so many such studies coming from a societal institution often known for its hostility to religion.

Pascal's Wager Revisited

To get the most out of church, get actively involved in it. As mentioned above, a big factor in enhancing well-being are the social networks formed there. And go at least once a week. Anything less often than that makes the wellness benefits fall off, as the Gallup survey referred to above attests. It underscores the importance of not being lukewarm in faith. And even if your heart is not yet into church, take your kids there if you have them. It will boost the odds of both you and them living longer, being happier, and staying out of trouble.

What about watching worship services online or on television, as has been commonly practiced since the Covid pandemic? Definitive studies on this haven't been published at the time of this writing, but Tyler VanderWeele of the Harvard T. H. Chan School of Public Health is confident the positive effect is smaller than that of in-person worship, largely because of the lack of the communal aspect and face-to-face contact.[17]

Finally, let's get something clear. You might say, "Wait a minute. I know lots of religious people in bad health, who've died fairly young, who are alcoholics, or who always feel miserable." And as regards the "niceness" factor discussed in chapter 16, you may say you know plenty of churchie folks who are anything but nice. Of course that's going to be the case. Remember, these are *averages*. These are *likelihoods*. Church-induced good health is not guaranteed. Lots of churchgoers die before their time, and plenty of atheists live long and fruitful lives — in the same way that being a fitness buff doesn't necessarily mean you'll outlive a chain-smoking couch-potato. On average, though, the health and longevity of religious persons exceed that of atheists, agnostics, and the lukewarm.

And this brings up the question: Would Christopher Hitchens have lived longer had he been a believer? A writer, commentator, and outspoken atheist, Hitchens died in 2011 at age 62 from throat cancer. If it was his drinking and smoking that killed him, turning toward God may not have quashed his penchant for alcohol and tobacco, but it may have eased it. Hitchens may well have lived longer had he been a practicing Christian. He should have taken Blaise Pascal's advice. The seventeenth-century French philosopher urged the nonreligious to make a wager. By embracing faith (he specifically had Christianity in mind) they would dramatically boost their chances of spending eternity in heaven after departing this world. By rejecting it they're taking the colossal risk of spending an eternity in hell. So it's best not to even entertain the latter eventuality.

Pascal's Wager doesn't just apply to the afterlife. As discussed in the pages to follow, rejecting faith risks misfortune in this life, while embracing it has body-and-mind rewards.

Chapter 1

BOLSTER YOUR BODILY HEALTH

Experts recommend a number of measures to improve your health and lengthen your life. They include (in no particular order): Eat healthy foods. Get regular exercise. Get seven to eight hours of sleep. Don't smoke. Get a college education. Get and stay married. Go to church regularly.

Come again? Regarding the last, how could sitting in a pew listening to a minister, priest, rabbi, or imam improve your health and longevity—especially when you could be out exercising Sunday morning instead? We normally associate good physical health with manifestly physical activities like eating healthy foods, not overeating, regular exercise, regular checkups, taking medicines, taking vitamins, washing hands, being safety-conscious, and good hygiene. Church seems like a sedentary activity. Well, for one thing, religious people tend to carry out these healthy practices to a greater extent than nonreligious people, even though religion typically doesn't even address them. Additionally, faith-filled folks are more often around others who remind them to get exercise, take their medicines, see the doctor, and steer clear of unhealthy habits.[1] This is because they're more likely to be married and not live alone, and have larger social support networks thanks to their church.

And that leads us to Vanessa's story. Since she was around nineteen, Vanessa had severe joint pain. Her lack of discipline and habit of procrastinating didn't help things. One day her pastor issued a challenge to read the Bible in ninety days. She resolved to do it. "In doing that I felt like something shifted in me. If I'm able to do this, what else am I capable of doing?" She stumbled upon a podcast on the importance of avoiding gluttony, of eating right, and exercising in order to take care of our bodies for the glory of God. "That was it for me…I decided I am done with being extremely tired all the time. I am done with being sick all the time. I am done with not having any energy. I am done with being overweight…I am working towards where God wants me to be." She started getting up at 5am to go to the gym and work out. "I'm eating better. My children are eating better. My children are seeing what I eat (e.g., fruits and vegetables) and want some of it and that's a blessing…I pray every time I take care of myself. I'm like, God I want to honor You with everything I have in me. I want to honor You with my mind. I want to honor You with my heart. I want to honor You with my spirit. I want to honor You with my physical being."[2]

Vanessa views her body as sacred and a gift from God. That's a big incentive to treat it as such. The Bible teaches that the body is a temple of the Holy Spirit (1 Corinthians 6:19), prompting many Christians to eat right and stay fit while steering clear of harmful things like booze, drugs, cigarettes, and risky sexual behaviors. Some religions or denominations forbid alcohol and tobacco, which may take some fun out of life but those believers get the last laugh with a longer life. Other faiths permit some of that fun, but stress doing so in moderation.

Take smoking for example. The faithful are much less likely to smoke and if they do, it's fewer cigarettes per day. In fact, someone who attends religious services weekly or more and prays and reads the Bible at least daily is 90 percent less likely to smoke than someone who doesn't do those things, according to Harold G. Koenig and colleagues at the Center for Spirituality, Theology and Health at Duke University Medical Center.[3]

This book's introduction lists various diseases to which churchgoers are less prone. Such ailments appear to have no relation to churchgoing. A case in point is meningococcal disease. A U.K. medical team investigated preventative measures against it, which causes meningitis and in some cases sepsis. It particularly affects those ages 16 through 21. After surveying some 144 youths in order to determine risk factors of getting the disease, the team found two big preventative measures: getting vaccinated, and church. Come again? What could church have to do with it? The most plausible explanation, say the study's authors, is "attendance at a religious event is associated with other lifestyle factors that promote health and protect against infection."[4]

In another study on acute-care patients at Duke University Medical Center, Koenig and David B. Larson revealed not only that churchgoers are seriously ill less often, but when they do get sick enough to be hospitalized they spend a lot less time there. "Unaffiliated (non-churchgoing) patients spent an average of 25 days in the hospital, compared with 11 days for affiliated patients."[5] What accounts for the difference? Medical illness is frequently accompanied by fear, uncertainty, and loss of control. When prolonged, depression and loss of hope can set in. As discussed in the next chapter, the mental literally affects the physical. But those who trust in God have an advantage. "We think that the single greatest impact that religion has on health is its ability to help patients cope with medical illness," said Koenig.[6] He told Dr. Laurie Marbas in a video interview, "It's a belief system that gives meaning to life, particularly when bad things happen. When people get sick, if they lose a loved one, if they go through severe trauma, that's when people start asking the questions, 'What is the meaning of life?', 'Why am I here?', 'Why did this happen?' People who have a strong religious faith, a strong connection with God, seem to be able to weather those events much better. They're able to find meaning more rapidly and integrate those experiences better."[7]

In addition to spending less time in the hospital, the faithful have better prospects of surviving. An Italian team studied the effects of religiosity on liver transplant patients. While they didn't measure frequency of church attendance, they determined that low-religiosity patients had lower post-transplant survival rates compared with those who engaged in such things as seeking God's help, trusting God, and trying to discern His will regarding their disease. One patient reported to the investigators, "I recovered my life by the will of someone up there who loves me. I knew I was in God's hands, I had great faith in Him, I was with Him. This closeness made me feel strong and calm." The investigators related that when faced with a serious physical illness, such patients "discover a new way of looking at themselves and explore inner aspects and spiritual horizons; this could create a sense of hope, new stimuli for the mind, and energy."[8]

As opposed to religious attendance engendering health and well-being, it has been suggested that religious institutions attract already-healthy people, including those who don't drink heavily or smoke and who already have strong social interactions. But health and well-being tend to improve among those who were struggling before they started attending church. "The analyses here indicate that attenders did not all start off with such good behaviors; to some extent, their good health behaviors and more extensive social relationships occurred in conjunction with attendance," write William Strawbridge of the Human Population Laboratory in Berkeley, Calif. along with three colleagues in their study, "Religious Attendance Increases Survival by Improving and Maintaining Good Health Behaviors, Mental Health, and Social Relationships."[9] Echoing that point are Ellen Idler and Stanislav Kasl of Rutgers and Yale respectively, who analyzed a twelve-year survey of older persons. They concluded churchgoing plays an independent role in better health outcomes that isn't accounted for by prior health status. It's thanks to "something which is apparently unique to the experience of attendance at religious services," they write. "Religious involvement appears to invigorate everyday life in the present, and to be a source of help for troubles in the future."[10]

Puzzling the Skeptics

Even with copious replication of the churchgoing-health findings, there was skepticism. This isn't surprising considering the intense secularism within academia. They criticized study methods and design. Rebuttals to those critics included claims they were overemphasizing the few negative findings while dismissing the many positive results, as well as misunderstanding epidemiological methods. Having reviewed more than 1,200 studies on religion and health, Harold Koenig and eight other colleagues penned an editorial in *The International Journal of Psychiatry in Medicine* observing that the vast majority of the studies revealed a positive relationship between religiosity and mental health, physical health, or lower use of health services. Particularly notable is that relatively few showed no relationship, and fewer still showed a negative relationship.[11] That was in 1999. Koenig estimates there now have been more than 6,000 studies on the religion/health relationship, and still, the vast majority indicate a positive one.[12]

On the question of whether churchgoing leads to good health rather than the other way around, another team of researchers, three with the Harvard T. H. Chan School of Public Health and one with Harvard Medical School, aimed to eliminate all doubt. They analyzed data from the ongoing Nurses' Health Study survey covering a twenty-year time span. To bullet-proof their methodology they were able to monitor if survey respondents reported attending religious services at certain points over the course of many years. This revealed whether the churchgoing preceded the health conditions, or vice-versa. Their findings were consistent with nearly every other study on this topic: it's churchgoing that causes better health and longer lives. "Attending a religious service more than once per week was associated with 33% lower all-cause mortality compared with women who had never attended religious services," they wrote. Attending once a week or less than weekly resulted in a 26 percent and 13 percent lower risk of all-cause mortality respectively. They noted that frequent attendance is associated with a significantly lower risk of cardiovascular- and cancer-related death—particularly breast cancer death. Their advice to caregivers is, "Our results do not imply that health care professionals should prescribe attendance at religious services, but for those who already hold religious beliefs, attendance at services could be encouraged as a form of meaningful social participation."[13]

Mitigating Mortality

Based on a review of several dozen studies, active worship enhances longevity mainly by helping to prevent healthy people from becoming sick or impaired, concluded Lynda Powell along with Leila Shahabi of the University of Miami and Carl Thoresen of Stanford. Church attendance, they wrote in their report, "confers some generalized type of protection against mortality."[14] But in an interview with *Newsweek*, Powell was less reserved. One thing "blew my socks off," she's quoted as saying. Regular churchgoers live longer than non-churchgoers; they have a 25 percent reduced risk of death. "This is really powerful," she intoned. The data mainly was based on studies of Christian populations, but she thinks the conclusions hold for any organized religion.[15]

Some years later, Powell along with Yoichi Chida and Andrew Steptoe conducted a study in which they systematically reviewed sixty-nine studies on the association between religion and longevity among initially healthy, and among diseased populations. This was a meta-analysis, which statistically evaluates most if not all of the available studies on a given subject and aggregates the results. Meta-analyses are important because they convey the overall consensus of studies, whereas individual studies could be subject to error. And the overall consensus in this case echoed Powell's earlier results. Among initially healthy people, religious attendance was associated with a 23 percent reduction in risk of early death.[16]

In a meta-analysis of forty-two studies on the subject, top researchers came to a similar conclusion, calculating that lower religious involvement carries a 29 percent higher risk of death.[17]

Kibbutzim in Contrast

Israel has a system of collective communities known as kibbutzim. They traditionally focused on agriculture but many now also produce a variety of goods. There are religious kibbutzim in which the members are devout Jews, and secular kibbutzim where the members typically are not so devout or they're nonreligious. Israeli scholars juxtaposed these communities to test religion's association with mortality. They monitored eleven religious and eleven secular kibbutzim over sixteen years. By the end of that period, 199 deaths had occurred in the secular kibbutzim and 69 in the religious ones. After controlling for various other factors there still was a "substantial excess rate of death" for members of secular kibbutzim. Reasons suggested for the devout Jews' lower mortality include higher emotional well-being derived from living in a cohesive religious community, prayer-induced relaxation, and stabler families.[18]

Lengthen Your Lifespan

What if you were told you can add several years to your life with no need to jog three miles a day, no need to give up your beloved chocolate, no need to survive on a diet of kale and fish, no need to swallow four capsules of anti-aging supplements each day, while still being able to scarf down those ketchup-drenched French fries once in a while? It sounds too good to be true. Well it isn't. Just stroll over to a nearby church each weekend. It's a mere one hour out of your 168-hour week. It also wouldn't hurt to throw in a Bible study or charity drive or two.

Skeptical? Lots of experts who study longevity were too, up until around the 1990s. That's when more and more studies came out showing the link between church and health. A 1999 investigation particularly made an impression among scholars and health professionals in terms of its thoroughness, ensuring no other factors were influencing the results.[19] In "Religious Involvement and U.S. Adult Mortality," Robert Hummer of the University of Texas at Austin along with fellow sociologists Richard Rogers, Charles Nam, and Christopher Ellison analyzed data from the National Health Interview Survey to gauge the effect of religious attendance on health/ mortality among older adults. Comparing participants' data with the follow-up period six years later, the researchers unearthed that people who never attend church have 1.87 times the risk of death compared with those who attend more than once a week. "This translates into a seven-year difference in life expectancy at age 20 between those who never attend and those who attend more than once a week," declared the authors.[20]

The study involved analyzing data on 21,204 people, of whom 2,016 had died by the end of the follow-up period. The scholars segmented the initial group into four categories according to frequency of religious attendance: never, less than once a week, weekly, and more than once a week. They estimated a 20-year-old weekly churchgoer is expected to live to age 82 (assuming, of course, he or she never stops attending), a more-than weekly churchgoer age 83, while a never-attender is expected to live to 75 ½. For a less-than-once-a-week attender life expectancy is 80. Those findings are startling enough. Even more striking, among African Americans the longevity difference between attending more than once a week and never attending is a whopping fourteen years; a life expectancy of 66 versus 80.

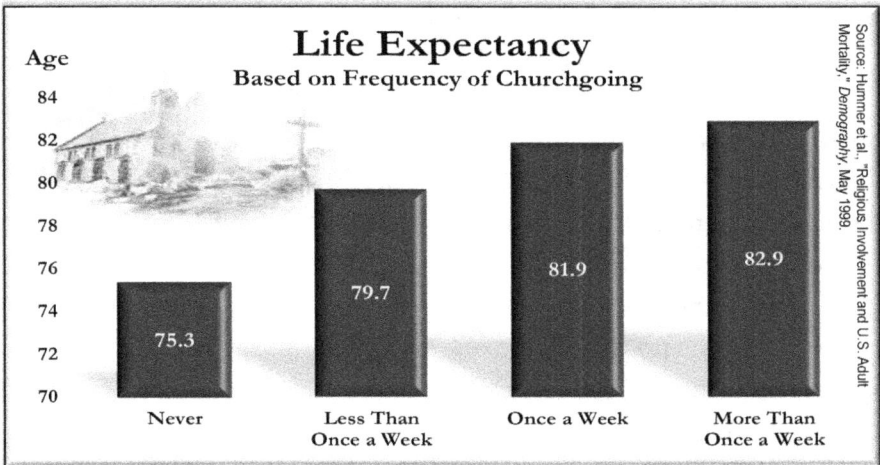

Life Expectancy
Based on Frequency of Churchgoing

Age

Never: 75.3
Less Than Once a Week: 79.7
Once a Week: 81.9
More Than Once a Week: 82.9

Source: Hummer et al., "Religious Involvement and U.S. Adult Mortality," *Demography*, May 1999.

Unmarried people who don't attend church "have especially high mortality" according to Hummer.[21] So if you're single, divorced, or widowed and not going to church, you're pushing your luck. While it isn't so easy to marry, it's easy to set aside an hour each Sunday morning for worship—since you're probably not doing much else then.

In addition to better health behavior, Hummer thinks it's the social interaction associated with church that mainly accounts for greater longevity. This is reflected in areas where mortality differences based on religious attendance is greatest: deaths from respiratory diseases, diabetes, and infectious diseases. Never-attenders are about *four times* more likely to die from these compared with more-than-once-a-week churchgoers. As the study authors point out, diabetes being among those causes of death hints at the importance of social aspects of churchgoing in extending lifespans, as family and friends often help diabetics maintain a regimented care program. And respiratory diseases being on the list suggests behavioral aspects stemming from public worship or lack thereof play a big role, such as smoking.

What about praying at home without going to church? Hummer says there's far weaker evidence for the positive effect of private religious activity on longevity.[22] This is in line with a recurring theme in this book: being spiritual without going to church doesn't produce the same earthly benefits.

The Hummer study shows that religious involvement is nearly as important as education in influencing longevity. A twenty-five-year-old male with a bachelor's degree can expect to live 9.3 years longer than a man with less than a high school education, according to the Centers for Disease Control and Prevention. For women the gap is 8.6 years.[23]

Hummer has no religious axe to grind. He wrote in a PowerPoint, "Robert Hummer does not claim a religious affiliation and would answer 'never' on questions regarding frequency of religious attendance and frequency of other religious-based activities." As to whether he recommends encouraging people to attend church just for the health benefits, he does not.[24]

The Longevity Project was a study that tracked about 1,500 people for more than eighty years starting in 1921 in an effort to determine what factors lead to longer life. In 2012 Howard Friedman and Leslie Martin published the results in their book *The Longevity Project*. Among women, the very religious tended to live longest and the least-religious the shortest. The latter "were generally bright and productive but they were less likely to be very extroverted and trusting, less likely to get and stay married, and less likely to have children or to be extensively involved in helping others," write Friedman and Martin. Helping others and other forms of social outreach are important for long life. Women who gradually stopped practicing their faith were at high risk if they also fell away from their community involvement.[25]

A more recent study, published in 2018, concluded that religiosity tacks on five to ten years to your life. Laura Wallace of Ohio State's department of psychology along with three other colleagues took a novel approach: analyzing obituaries. As critics have alleged that the traditional methodology of self-reporting in surveys has been open to the possibility of error, Wallace and her team believe their data-gathering technique eliminates that. The mention of a religious affiliation in the obituary told them who the likely churchgoers were. They did two analyses: on 505 obits from the *Des Moines Register*, and 1,096 of them in forty-two major newspapers from throughout the United States.

If you live in Des Moines and pray in the pews, you're golden. The deceased whose obituaries mentioned a church connection lived an average of 9.5 years longer than those whose did not. Even controlling for the effects of gender and marital status, the faithful lived 6.5 years longer. For their second survey nationwide, those indicating religiosity lived 5.6 years longer. And what are some of the factors behind the good news for churchgoing? "Many religions promote stress reducing practices that may improve health such as gratitude, prayer, or meditation," observed the study team. "Religious belief may also provide people with a sense that the world is predictable, which should make them feel more in control of their outcomes and thus reduce anxiety associated with believing the world is unpredictable."[26]

Other studies have found varying numbers of additional years of life for churchgoers. At the low end is 1.8 to 3.1 years as calculated by Daniel Hall of the University of Pittsburgh Medical Centers. And still, that's a better deal than Lipitor. He estimated churchgoing adds about the same number of years to your life as that wonder drug, at a cheaper cost.[27]

You could take Lipitor to lengthen your lifespan, and you could jog two miles every other day, which also adds about three years.[28] But instead of panting and gasping four times a week in the heat, cold, and rain, why not add even more years by relaxing once a week in a nice, cozy pew? Or, do both for double the impact.

Heart of the Matter

Prayer provides comfort and hope; it's comforting to know you're not only loved by God but are being prayed for by others. That not only warms the heart, it helps make you heart-healthy. Those who pray often and regularly go to church have a 40 percent lower likelihood of diastolic hypertension (high blood pressure) than their non-churchgoing and infrequently praying counterparts, according to a team of six M.D.'s and Ph.D.'s.[29] Another six-member study team led by David Larson of Duke disclosed that for men over fifty-five, mean diastolic pressure is about 6mm lower and mean systolic pressure almost 9mm lower among weekly church attenders who consider religion highly important, compared with the non-religious. This is quite significant, intone the investigators, because for the overall population, even a 2 to 4mm Hg reduction in mean blood pressure can bring down cardiovascular disease by 10 to 20 percent. The good news for non-churchgoing non-smokers is that there was little difference in blood pressure between high and low religious groups. But among smokers, "risk of an abnormal diastolic pressure for low attenders was almost 4 times higher and abnormal systolic twice as high as for high attenders."

This is noteworthy for another reason. It has been suggested churchgoers enjoy better health because of less smoking, drinking, and unhealthy eating. In this study, however, it was among smokers that religious observance influenced the large difference in blood pressure. So it isn't necessarily the absence of smoking and other unhealthy behaviors that lead to better health. Larson and colleagues suggested it may reflect a moderating effect of religion on blood pressure, stemming from religion's encouragement of positive relationships, resulting in less stress and anxiety.[30]

Marino Bruce of the Center for Research on Men's Health at Vanderbilt University along with ten colleagues from various institutions confirmed that frequent church attendance is associated with greater longevity in addition to less stress. Compared with those attending church at least monthly, non-churchgoers had significantly higher systolic blood pressure, HDL cholesterol, and total cholesterol/HDL. The relationship still held after adjusting for education, poverty status, health insurance status, self-rated health, and social support, pointing to strong evidence that active worship independently affects mortality. Those attending church more than weekly had a 49 percent unadjusted reduced risk for all-cause mortality (46 percent reduced risk after adjusting for age, sex, race, and chronic medical conditions). "Health benefits of religiosity may also be attributed, in part, to its impact on two less commonly cited domains, compassion and a sense of holiness," write Bruce and colleagues. "Holiness gives meaning and purpose to life and inspires commitment to something greater than self. Holiness instills love, joy, peace, hope and fulfillment, fosters a sense of inter-connectedness with others, promotes a sense of wholeness in life, and engenders a greater personal relationship with a higher power, possibly explaining the health benefits attributed to religiosity."[31]

As mentioned in the introduction, Byron Johnson (then of UPenn, now of Baylor) and colleagues reviewed nearly 800 studies related to the influence of religion on health and social outcomes, the vast majority of which found positive influences. They lay out the findings in *Objective Hope: Assessing the Effectiveness of Faith-Based Organizations* (henceforth Objective Hope). Of 29 studies addressing hypertension, 22 affirmed that religious involvement benefits the heart. Six studies found no association and just one was negative.[32] In Harold Koenig's systematic review, among the highest-quality studies, 62 percent reported significantly lower hypertension among those who are more religious.[33]

Decreased Disability

Following are highlights from a tiny sample of the many, many studies showing religion's positive relationship with health and longevity:

- A twelve-year study found that frequent churchgoers as a whole are significantly less physically disabled than infrequent attenders. Churchgoers scored better on physical activity, smoking, depression, alcohol use, friendship, family ties, social activities, holiday celebrations, and optimism. Religious attendance was "a kind of lynchpin" connecting them to friends, relatives, holiday celebrations, and other social activities. Worshipping may among other things bring a person to a transcendent state in which the body and its disabilities don't matter much to that person, which ironically could speed recovery from disability. These findings come from a study by Idler and Kasl of 2,812 older adults.[34]

- Based on a survey of about 2,000 older persons in Marin County, Calif., frequent church attenders were less likely to smoke, exercised more, had more friends and social contacts, and stayed married to a greater extent. At the end of the five-year study period the death rate was 21 per 1,000 for weekly church attenders, 25 per 1,000 for occasional attenders, and 32 per 1,000 for non-attenders.[35] Similar results were found in a study done in Alameda County, Calif. on 5,000 residents over the course of twenty-eight years.[36] And among Mexican Americans sixty-five and older, based on an eight-year follow-up period, weekly churchgoers had a 32 percent lower risk of death compared with never-attenders.[37]

- An eight-year effort in Taiwan monitored 3,739 persons age fifty-three and above, finding that those who frequently practice their faith have the longest life expectancy. This held whether it was public or private worship. Buddhism for example often involves private meditation, prayer, and/or incense-burning. Based on this, the researchers concluded religion positively influences health not just from social interaction but from other factors relating to private prayer and meditation. Interestingly, life expectancy of those having no religious affiliation was above that of believers who "never" or "rarely" practiced their faith—but not as high as those categorized as "sometimes."[38]

• Wei Zhang of the University of Hawaii at Manoa studied the very elderly in China—ages 80 to 105—finding "religious participation to be significantly associated with lower risk of mortality for oldest (of the) old women and for individuals in poor health." Exercise and leisure activities partially accounted for this association, which suggests religious participation boosts longevity among Chinese when it's combined with other socially integrated and cognitively stimulating activities.[39]

Church cuts down on cancer. In one of the many studies on this subject, a research team looked at religious practice and cancer rates by U.S. county. Rates are lower where there's high religious membership among the population, particularly lower among more conservative denominations.[40]

Religiosity surprisingly is associated with a higher body mass index. However, the 2020 meta-analysis revealing this also found it's associated with lower blood pressure, cholesterol, stress, and inflammation, along with fewer heart attacks and better vascular health.[41]

Health Benefits of Fasting

In all major religions, the devout are known to fast for their spiritual health. What's remarkable is how good fasting is for physical and mental health. It may involve skipping a meal or all meals for a given day, reducing food intake per meal, or spurning food for multiple consecutive days.

Reasons for fasting include: to voluntarily do something arduous solely for the purpose of demonstrating to God faith in, love for, and commitment to Him; to fortify one's prayers and petitions by showing God a willingness to even suffer for Him and communicate how strongly one feels about a petition or desire; to atone for one's sins and/or the sins of others; to focus one's mind on the spiritual rather than on things of the world; and to instill self-discipline in order to build character, patience, and other virtues.

Much research has been done on the many health benefits of fasting. It is said to improve blood sugar control, fight chronic inflammation, lower blood pressure, lower cholesterol, prevent neurodegenerative disorders, aid in weight loss (obviously), extend longevity, and fight cancer.[42] Fasting for two to three days—maybe even shorter durations—can reset the entire immune system.[43]

Religious adherents also may fast from treats and comforts such as sweets, car air conditioning, or hot water. The last involves taking cold showers. Research has shown cold showers boost immunity and circulation, improve hair and skin, help weight loss, boost testosterone (for men), drain the lymphatic system, and improve body temperature regulation. That cold blast of water also improves mental health: it boosts alertness and mood, increases willpower, and last but not least, alleviates depression. Those with heart conditions, however, should be careful. Cold water immersion has been known to prompt heart attacks.[44]

Helping the Poor and Disadvantaged

Tremendous benefits of church flow to those of low income, poor health, and/or low education. A study focusing on elderly poor confirmed that churchgoers among them lived longer.[45] The churchgoing poor are more likely to have social connectedness as well as "a coherent belief system that may allay feelings of isolation, low control, and despair and improve one's sense of self-efficacy," write

Powell, Shahabi, and Thoresen in their meta-analysis "Religion and Spirituality: Linkages to Physical Health."[46]

Another benefit is material support. Churches provide resources not readily available elsewhere which may include goods, services, shelter, and counseling, as well as housing, financial, and medical assistance. Regarding the last, Objective Hope found that church-based hypertension intervention programs have been successful in lowering blood pressure within African American congregations. A church-sponsored telephone counseling program for Latina, Black, and White women in Los Angeles helped maintain the practice of getting mammograms, reducing the nonadherence rate from 23 percent to 16 percent. Elsewhere, an intensive church-based cancer control outreach program had a substantial positive effect on the awareness and behavior of under-screened Hispanic women. Of the 25 studies reviewed by Objective Hope on health-related interventions administered by faith-based groups, 23 had beneficial outcomes. Just two found no association, and no study determined a negative impact.[47]

Chapter 2

THE PSYCHO-SOCIAL
AFFECTS THE PHYSICAL

With a mindset that the body is a temple of the Holy Spirit, churchgoers strive to take practical, concrete steps to improve their health. There are more subtle benefits as well. It's commonly known that social interaction improves both mental and physical health; so does having a positive self-image. And good coping skills ease stressful events such as illness and grief. Other psycho-social factors that improve the physical include having a meaningful and coherent worldview as well as a strong marriage and harmonious family life. Churchgoing fosters all of these, which in turn foster longevity.

Aristotle's dictum that humans are social animals is almost a cliche. People need social interaction, and churches help provide that. Anthropologists say we succeeded as a species—rose to the top of the food chain, if you will—because of our ability to cooperate in order to hunt game, protect ourselves from predators, and survive in difficult natural environments. Jared Diamond, author of *The World Until Yesterday: What Can We Learn from Traditional Societies?*, spent years living with pre-modern tribes in Papua New Guinea—the types of societies constituting most of human existence. He observed that the people constantly are engaged in conversation and hardly ever are alone.[1] That helps explain why they experience very low rates of clinical depression. Given humans' roots in social interaction it's no surprise that in our modern world this helps engender healthier, happier, and more productive lives. But all too often people are socially isolated, far removed from the interaction typical of pre-modern societies. Loneliness and anxiety are pervasive. Things get even worse under pandemic-related seclusion.

Opportunities for friendship and fellowship do much to alleviate isolation and consequent anxiety. People feel more relaxed and less stressed. This in turn positively affects health. Clubs and other organizations facilitate group interaction; places of worship are especially good venues not only because of being with a group but also being with others who share the same belief system. Church social and educational activities include Bible study, dinner groups, discussion groups, lectures and talks, choir singing, ushering, greeting, charitable activities, religious education, committees and boards, youth groups and the like, which promote interaction, friendship, and communication.

"Christ gave me community," related Clay. "I have never felt more welcomed in any community than in the community of Christ. It took me two years to find a church after I started my journey to Christ, but once I did, the relationships I formed there stick with me to this day. I met my wife and my closest friends through church. How did I, someone who couldn't make friends to save his life just a year or two before, manage to find it in me to pursue close friendships? I knew that I had a spiritual bloodline in common with the people at my church. That motivated me to get to know them and to share life with them. Without that connection, I never would have tried."[2]

Clay may very well get more than he bargained for thanks to his newfound community. While a larger number of secular close friendships are associated with life satisfaction, church friendships result in even greater satisfaction. "Our findings suggest that a strong sense of religious identity may be the key factor setting congregational friendship apart from other social networks," write the University of Wisconsin's Chaeyoon Lim and Harvard's Robert Putnam in their study "Religion, Social Networks, and Life Satisfaction." However, they also conclude that when a person attends church yet doesn't consider religion to be very important to his or her sense of self, then church-connected friendships don't have that same effect on life satisfaction. That's why it's key be strong in faith or "intrinsically" religious (see chapter 12). Also of note, the researchers' analysis suggests that life satisfaction of churchgoers who have no friends at church isn't even as high as non-attenders' life satisfaction. This is hard to believe vis-à-vis the highly religious, who only care about having a close relationship with God. But it certainly is plausible with regard to churchgoers lukewarm in their faith.[3]

A study published in *Psychosomatic Medicine* confirmed that social interaction and religion prolong life. Thomas Oxman and Daniel Freeman of Dartmouth Medical School along with Eric Manheimer of the University of Texas Medical Branch examined the impact of social support and religion on the survival of 232 open-heart surgery patients at Dartmouth-Hitchcock Medical Center. Out of the forty-nine patients who reported they derived no strength and comfort from religion and who didn't participate in organized groups, ten died within six months after surgery. Of the seventy-two who did get religious strength and comfort and who were active in community, only two had died. That group's likelihood of survival was an astounding 14 times higher than the nonreligious/non-socially active.

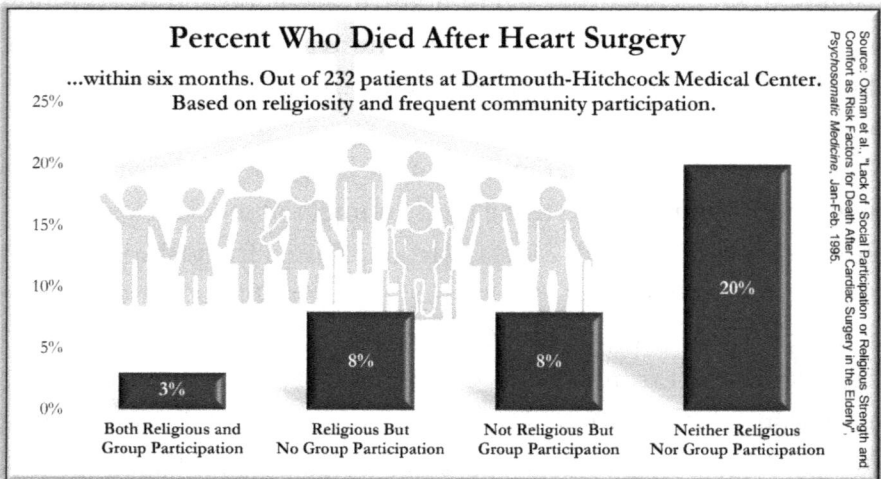

Percent Who Died After Heart Surgery

...within six months. Out of 232 patients at Dartmouth-Hitchcock Medical Center. Based on religiosity and frequent community participation.

Both Religious and Group Participation	Religious But No Group Participation	Not Religious But Group Participation	Neither Religious Nor Group Participation
3%	8%	8%	20%

Source: Oxman et al., "Lack of Social Participation or Religious Strength and Comfort as Risk Factors for Death After Cardiac Surgery in the Elderly", *Psychosomatic Medicine*, Jan-Feb. 1995.

The latter persons also are less likely to be married and have fewer emotionally close friends or family. Another noteworthy finding: social and religious factors have a bigger impact on mortality than do personality or mood. The authors suggest that physicians make simple inquiries about group participation and religious involvement "as routinely as they inquire and advise about cigarette smoking and hypertension." While doctors may have a hard time convincing patients to join religious or social groups, "asking about such behaviors and positively reinforcing them are unlikely to do serious harm, may improve quality of life, and in some cases may prove to be one final, useful bit of evidence that patients will use to alter their survival behaviors."[4]

Eran Shor of McGill University and David Roelfs of the University of Louisville sought to determine if health effects of religion stem from religious practices themselves or from the social aspect. So in a meta-analysis they looked at participation in both religious and nonreligious groups, concluding churchgoing isn't a uniquely beneficial form of social participation; lifetimes can be lengthened by regular involvement in other social settings, which may include card games, bingo, clubs and organizations, political activities, volunteerism, and family activities such as birthdays and celebrations. Their results showed that compared with a frequent churchgoer, mortality risk is 32 percent higher for someone with low religious participation. A person with low participation in nonreligious social settings has a 25 percent higher risk of death than the socially active. But the investigators say the 32 versus 25 percent difference isn't statistically significant. "Being part of a social group helps individuals gain and maintain helpful social relationships, provides them with an opportunity to engage in activities that they see as productive, and gives them a sense of purpose and self-worth."[5]

But can bingo or card games bestow the same sense of meaning and purpose as deep religious devotion? At church, people feel a connection to the divine and a higher power—something hard to replicate at a game of Texas hold'em. Touched on above are aspects of meaning and purpose that only religious involvement can confer. The rest of this book highlights numerous findings echoing those points, with proven effects on happiness and good health. One such finding was by scholars at the London School of Economics and the Erasmus University Medical Center in the Netherlands, who analyzed data on 9,000 middle-aged people and older in ten European countries. Among those with depression, being active in a religious organization was the only form of social engagement associated with a decline in depression four years later. Though they hypothesized that participation in nonreligious charitable organizations, social clubs, sports, community groups, political activities, and other types of social interaction would reduce depression, their results didn't show that. "Participation in religious organizations may offer mental health benefits beyond those offered by other forms of social participation," they concluded. In fact, "increased participation in political/community organizations was associated with higher depressive symptom scores."[6] So much for politics.

Social interaction coupled with spirituality definitely makes a difference, argues Baylor University epidemiologist Jeff Levin, author of *God, Faith, and Health: Exploring the Spirituality-Healing Connection*. He observes, "Religious fellowship is by itself a salient factor against illness. But when it comes to one's spiritual life, meaning it from the heart is the best protection of all."[7]

Purpose, Meaning, and Optimism

Religion is known for instilling a sense of purpose in life. That, in turn, lengthens life. A study led by Patricia Boyle of Rush University Medical Center surveyed more than 1,200 elderly, following up five years later to record who had died. Survey respondents who indicated they had a strong sense of purpose were about half as likely to pass away during those five years.[8] They also were less susceptible to Alzheimer's; those who scored in the ninetieth percentile on a purpose-of-life scale were 2.4 times likelier to avoid that dreaded disease than those scoring in the tenth percentile.[9]

A sense of meaning and purpose, especially in connection with devotion to God, boosts optimism which in turn boosts health. This particularly holds true for African Americans. Analyzing a survey of 1,126 older Blacks and Whites, Neal Krause of the University of Michigan found that Blacks are more likely to enjoy health-related benefits of religion. This may be because their congregations tend to be more cohesive, with greater spiritual and emotional support for worshipers. It leads to a more personal relationship with and feeling of connectedness to God, boosting optimism.[10]

Faith-powered hope and optimism are especially important in harrowing life-or-death situations. Whether it be war prisoners or political prisoners undergoing torture and deprivation, being lost in the wilderness, lost at sea, or overcoming a ghastly injury or disease, there are countless stories of people pulling through because of their trust in God.

Molecules of Emotion

When UPenn's Andrew Newberg conducted real-time brain scans on Franciscan nuns engaged in deep prayer, he saw many visible changes going on. "This was very exciting to us. We were actually looking at evidence that prayer has a measurable effect on the human brain. This is the kind of moment that a scientist lives for, and for me personally, it was a moment that both validated my interest in the spiritual brain and ignited my passion to learn much more." Newberg's work shows that praying is different from just thinking. Praying has unique and measurable physical effects within the brain.[11] That, in turn, positively affects the body as a whole.

Prayer and religion inspire hope, optimism, calmness, and tranquility that literally improve physical health. This involves hormones and the nervous system. Thoughts affect neurotransmitters, which are chemical messengers that transmit signals from brain cells to other cells including muscle and gland cells. A type of neurotransmitter are catecholamines, which include the stress hormones epinephrine (a.k.a. adrenaline) and norepinephrine. Sometimes called molecules of emotion, these chemicals are essential to prepare the body for stressful situations, i.e. "fight-or-flight" responses such as elevating the heart rate in order to be more physically capable when confronted with danger. Cortisol is another such hormone.

An absence of hope and optimism—which often results from an absence of church and prayer—can lead to chronically elevated levels of these chemicals, which increase blood pressure and suppress the immune system.[12]

Church and prayer also boost "parasympathetic" activities which include secreting saliva or digestive enzymes associated with tranquil situations, thus lowering blood pressure. To help achieve this, Christian psychotherapist Charles Zeiders recommends repeatedly uttering the Jesus Prayer which goes, "Lord Jesus Christ, son of the living God, have mercy on me, a sinner."[13] It's often recited throughout the day—typically very slowly, verbally or mentally—by those taking to heart St. Paul's exhortation in the Bible to "pray without ceasing." (1 Thessalonians 5:17)

Another factor is lower inflammatory cytokine levels. Cytokines are proteins that cells release to affect the behavior of other cells. Inflammatory cytokines tend to produce inflammation, fever, or tissue destruction. Inflammation can be good in that white blood cells attack microscopic invaders, but too much of certain types of inflammation lead to a variety of ills such as cancer, diabetes, cardiovascular disease, arthritis, and asthma. Prolonged inflammation causes atherosclerosis—i.e. the accumulation of fatty deposits along the lining of arteries—which increases the risk of heart attack and stroke.[14] Negative emotions such as anger, unforgiveness, insecurity, and lack of a sense of meaning are associated with higher levels of inflammatory cytokines. Positive emotions and attitudes such as awe, empathy, forgiveness, contentment, and meaning/purpose tend to elicit lower levels.[15] As discussed throughout this book, active worship nourishes these emotions and attitudes.

This even could impact your chances of surviving a pandemic. In the case of Covid, the most common killer is ARDS or adult respiratory distress syndrome which occurs when cytokine levels surpass a critical threshold during a "cytokine storm." Previously elevated levels of cytokines bring that threshold into greater reach (see chart). So it's crucial to maintain lower levels. David Hanscom, an orthopedic surgeon who now focuses on alleviating chronic mental and physical pain, writes in *Psychology Today* of several ways to do that. They include exercising, eliminating anxiety, practicing forgiveness, halting negative talk, and being nice.[16]

With the possible exception of exercising, all of those are part and parcel of religious devotion.

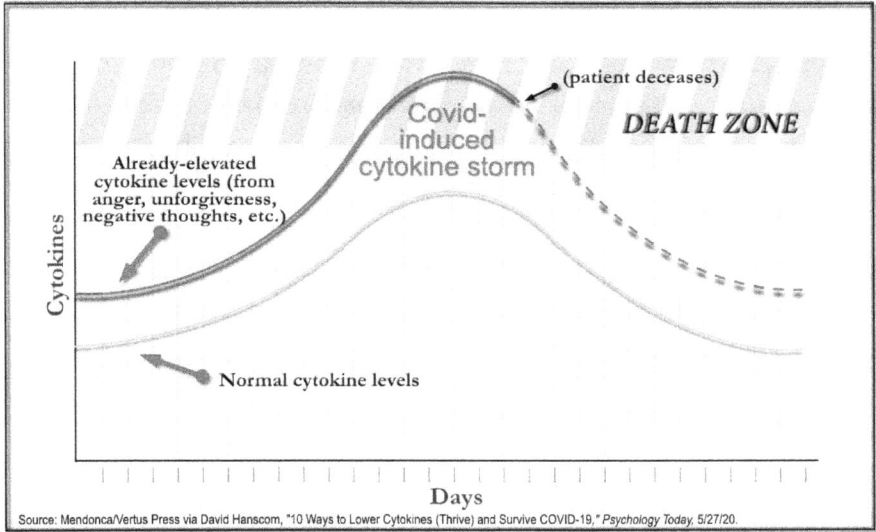

Source: Mendonca/Vertus Press via David Hanscom, "10 Ways to Lower Cytokines (Thrive) and Survive COVID-19," *Psychology Today*, 5/27/20.

"From cutting-edge research in new fields such as psychophysiology and psychoneuroimmunology, we have learned that emotions are 'hardwired' into our autonomic nervous, endocrine, and immune systems," writes Jeff Levin in *God, Faith, and Health*. "As a consequence, what we feel can affect the physiological functioning of our bodies...Whatever elicits heartfelt emotional responses is a potentially protective factor, epidemiologically speaking...In this regard, religious worship has few equivalents."[17] Levin observes that feelings of love for God, as well as feeling loved by God, are associated with higher self-esteem and self-mastery, and less depression, all of which affect the physical. He points to evidence reviewed by Michael McCullough of (at that time) Southern Methodist University indicating that the emotional benefits of prayer lead to neuroimmunological and cardiovascular changes that can improve health.[18]

In Koenig's systematic review, 23 of 31 studies found significantly lower levels of stress hormones (such as cortisol, epinephrine, and norepinephrine) in more religious persons as well as in patients receiving spiritual interventions.[19]

Giving generously also has its bodily rewards. Autoimmune disorders take place when the immune system mistakenly attacks healthy tissues. Such diseases include rheumatoid arthritis, type 1 diabetes, and lupus. T-suppressor cells move about the body help-ing to ensure that such immune overreactions don't occur. A study was done comparing the level of T-suppressor cells between those who gave 9 percent or more of their annual income to their church, and those who gave 2 percent or less. The more generous givers had higher levels of T-suppressor cells, thus greater protection from autoimmune disorders. The stingier givers also had poorer scores on church attendance, stress-coping, forgiveness, and hostility.[20]

To Forgive is Divine

When Ryan was fourteen he found out his dad was living a double life, having an affair. "Because of my teenage immaturity and my anger towards my dad, I started rebelling. I got in with a rowdy group of friends and we would go out and do destructive things." A few years later, Ryan began drinking heavily. "I'd drink and smoke until I passed out. I hit the lowest point of my life…I started wondering, is this the meaning of life, is there a purpose for my life? It was at that moment where I knew that I needed God, and I would start looking up YouTube videos about heaven, about hell, about Jesus, about God—I started hearing these testimonies from people who went through similar things that I went through. They ended up living totally new, amazing lives with Jesus Christ. I got on my knees, and it was at that moment where I experienced this heavy weight lifted off of my shoulders. I began reading the Bible. All the questions that I had in life were being answered by the Bi-ble, by the Word of God…I wrote a letter to my dad and I told him that I had forgiven him because Christ forgave me, and I asked for forgiveness as well for all of the things that I did. And I was able to forgive all of the people that have hurt me in the past because of the forgiveness that I received through Jesus Christ. He has filled all the voids in my heart. He has given me peace, love, joy, contentment. He's given me a plan and a purpose."[21]

What's the best medicine for anger and grudges? Forgiveness. Not only is it obvious in personal stories like Ryan's, it's the growing consensus among researchers. There's strong empirical evidence that forgiveness boosts overall life satisfaction, positive emotions, and social support—and reduces or eliminates depression, hostility, anxiety, substance abuse, and nicotine dependence.[22] It reduces infection, to boot. A study revealed that persons unable to forgive themselves, forgive others, or feel forgiven by God were more likely to have had an infection during the month prior to being surveyed. This is particularly important in the context of pandemic. As stated in *Crossroads*, the newsletter of Duke University's Center for Spirituality, Theology and Health, "These findings underscore the importance of having a strong religious faith and having positive interactions within one's religious community in order to boost resilience to this dreaded virus (and other flu viruses as well)."[23]

Fred Luskin, director of the Stanford University Forgiveness Projects, explains in his book *Forgive for Good* that based on many scientific studies, more forgiving people have less stress and fewer health problems, including lower susceptibility to heart disease and cancer. He writes that lack of forgiveness negatively affects blood pressure, muscle tension, and immune response. Holding a grudge for an extended period of time can damage the heart and blood vessels. High levels of anger can make a person three times more likely to get heart disease. This is because of the above-mentioned stress chemicals which cause a narrowing of coronary and peripheral arteries and affect heart function. Luskin described sessions he conducted in which participants received instruction on forgiveness. Thanks to the training they suffered less both emotionally and physically after forgiving others. Personal rewards included a reduction or elimination of stress, stress-related backaches, stomach aches, and insomnia.[24]

Not forgiving someone may hurt that someone in several ways including emotionally, situationally, or reputationally. If the non-forgiver is you, that may be precisely what you want: to inflict a form of revenge or punishment on the alleged wrongdoer. This may bring a certain feeling of satisfaction. But you're ultimately hurting yourself. Holding a grudge and stewing with thoughts of revenge can come back to bite you in the form of higher stress, anxiety, hostility, anger, depression, substance abuse, and/or health problems like high blood pressure. Excess molecules of (negative) emotion adversely affect blood pressure and cholesterol levels. Slow burns, or long-term low-level anger, can mean a constant release of them. You may be so used to it that you don't even realize it's abnormal.

> "Gladness of heart is the very life of a person, and
>   cheerfulness prolongs his days...Envy and an-
>   ger shorten one's days, and anxiety brings on
>   premature old age." (Sirach 30:22,24)

Men under fifty-five and prone to anger are three times more likely to get early-onset heart disease and five times more likely to have a heart attack. That's based on a Johns Hopkins study in which researchers analyzed records of 1,055 men who were kept track of for 32 to 48 years. Anger is an even bigger predictor of heart disease than hypertension and diabetes, they found.[25] Another study, where researchers monitored about 13,000 men and women enrolled in the Atherosclerosis Risk In Communities Study, showed a nearly three-fold higher risk of heart attack among those prone to anger.[26]

Learning to forgive as directed by your religion aids in avoiding these negatives and leads to reconciliation and better relationships. Strong belief in a higher power helps enable acceptance of unfortunate events and of alleged perpetrators by trusting that the bad as well as the good are part of a grand plan. Multiple studies, including one by Daniel Escher of the University of Notre Dame's sociology department, have confirmed that when you sense God has forgiven you, it's easier to forgive both yourself and others. His study also verified that kids raised in faith are more prone to forgive later in life. And people who abandon their faith are less likely to forgive themselves and others. Observes Escher, "What seems to matter in promoting forgiveness, then, is that a person adheres to a religion or denomination; on the whole, the religiously unaffiliated have less of a propensity to forgive."[27]

Praying for a person helps you forgive that person. Attesting to this is a study by Florida State psychology professor Nathanial Lambert and colleagues. They divided undergraduate students into three groups. Every day for weeks, each participant in one group had to pray for a friend who had committed some offense against him or her. For another group, instead of praying, the participants had to think positive thoughts about a friend. A third group was directed to simply pray in general. The result: scoring highest on forgiveness were those who prayed for their friend. They also had a higher level of selfless concern.[28]

Ditch the grudges. Learning to forgive diminishes depression and boosts mental well-being. For more proof, consider the work of UM-Ann Arbor's Neal Krause and (at that time) UT Austin's Christopher Ellison. With a survey of 1,500 adults, they juxtaposed two types of forgivers: people who forgive on the condition that their alleged transgressors make amends or acts of restitution, and people who forgive unconditionally. Sure enough, unconditional forgivers have less psychological distress than conditional forgivers. With echoes of the Parable of the Unforgiving Servant (described below), many of the research subjects felt that God forgiving them for their own misdeeds makes them duty-bound to forgive others unconditionally. Krause and Ellison cited a man who remarked, "He forgives you for all things, regardless … and if He forgives, I most certainly can forgive." He added that he must do so unconditionally. Another man said failure to forgive is "almost an unpardonable sin." Not only do unconditional forgivers enjoy a greater sense of well-being, but based on Krause's and Ellison's findings, conditional forgivers and non-forgivers have more anxiety about dying. So forgiving makes you both happier and more accepting of the inevitable: death.[29]

Forgiving is hard. To bring yourself to do it you need every tool at your disposal. Without religion, it's doable. With religion, it's a lot more doable. Every major faith tradition teaches forgiveness. One of the most commonly recited prayers in Christianity, The Lord's Prayer, contains the lines "And forgive us our trespasses, as we forgive those who trespass against us." (Matthew 6:12) People spout off those lines without even thinking about them. But occasionally they're taken to heart. They tie in with the Parable of the Unforgiving Servant (Matthew 18:23-35). After a servant pleads with his king to forgive his unpayable debt, the king has compassion and does so. But afterward, the servant refuses to forgive the debt of a fellow servant. When the king finds out, he's justifiably appalled and throws the scoundrel into prison. The overarching lesson: if you don't forgive others, God won't forgive you. In that same Gospel, Peter asks Jesus how many times he should forgive someone when that someone sins again him. Peter suggests, seven times? Jesus responds, seventy times seven times. (Matthew 18:21-22)

Many passages of the Koran teach forgiveness. They include: "Hold to forgiveness, command what is right, and turn away from the ignorant." (Qur'an, 7: 199); "… They should rather pardon and overlook. Would you not love Allah to forgive you? Allah is Ever-Forgiving, Most Merciful." (Qur'an, 24:22); "The repayment of a bad action is one equivalent to it. But if someone pardons and puts things right, his reward is with Allah…" (Qur'an, 42:40); "… But if you pardon and exonerate and forgive, Allah is Ever-Forgiving, Most Merciful." (Qur'an, 64: 14)[30]

In addition to outright teachings, religion promotes forgiveness in other ways. "Perhaps specific aspects of the congregational climate, such as the overall level of expressiveness, empathy, and social concern among church members, may contribute to a parishioner's willingness to forgive," write Krause and Ellison.[31] This is one reason why organized religion—as opposed to mere spirituality—is associated with boosting forgiveness to a greater extent, according to another study. However, self-forgiveness is more associated with spirituality.[32]

Two types of forgiveness are decisional forgiveness and emotional forgiveness. Decisional forgiveness is an act of the will. It's the decision to forgive someone even though you're still harboring negative emotions like bitterness, hostility, and anger. Emotional forgiveness is when those feelings subside, replaced by neutral or positive feelings toward the person. Emotional forgiveness may eventually happen with or without decisional forgiveness, but decisional typically speeds the process of emotional forgiveness. So work on decisional forgiveness. Other types of forgiveness are self-forgiveness, and divine forgiveness, when you feel God has forgiven you.[33] Ask any Catholic coming out of the confession booth, and it's almost a sure bet they'll feel that way.

Alternative to Opioids

With much fanfare, prescription opioids came on the scene as a modern-day solution to conquer chronic pain. But there was a problem: millions of people were getting addicted, and tens of thousands dying from overdoses. The situation got so bad that federal health authorities called on doctors to dramatically cut back prescribing these siren songs. As an alternative, authorities encouraged non-drug solutions to manage pain including mindfulness meditation, yoga, massage therapy, acupuncture, and cognitive behavioral therapy.[34] Alas, they left out another promising alternative: prayer and religiosity.

In their paper "Spirituality/Religion and Pain," Christina Rush, Kaitlyn Vagnini, and Amy Wachholtz of the University of Colorado Denver psychology department write, "When carefully navigated, S/R (spirituality/religion) approaches may, in some cases, bring increased mastery over pain without any of the deleterious risks associated with opioid medications." Perceiving the presence of a loving and powerful being can instill a sense of safety and hope, helping a person transcend suffering. Religion tends to boost pain tolerance and even mitigate it. The authors cite a study comparing secular meditation with spiritual meditation involving migraine sufferers. The spiritual meditators had fewer migraines, lower anxiety, and greater pain tolerance.[35] Rush and colleagues also referred to an Iranian study in which two groups of migraine patients received equal doses of medicine for three months, but one group had a weekly, forty-five-minute session of intercessory prayer. The prayer group had significantly less pain at the end of the study period.[36] In another study, an image of the Blessed Virgin Mary was shown to practicing Catholics and a secular image (da Vinci's "Lady with an Ermine") to atheists and agnostics, who were administered painful electrical stimulations to the hand. Only the religious participants felt decreased pain.[37]

Even when the pain persists, religion can turn it into something meaningful, making it more bearable and even a source of happiness. In the Catholic tradition is the practice of offering up one's suffering to God, known as redemptive suffering. Moses fasted for forty days to atone for and appease God for the sins of His chosen people, the Israelites. Jesus sacrificed his earthly life to the Father to atone for the sins of humankind. In the same way, people unite their voluntary and involuntary sufferings with Jesus on the cross to atone for both their own sins and the sins of others. Just as God the Father was moved by the actions of Moses and Jesus, He's moved when people in pain pray that their sufferings are put toward a good spiritual purpose.

When he visits hospitals and nursing homes, Catholic priest and popular speaker Father John Riccardo prays with patients and asks them to offer up their sufferings for the benefit of others. He gives them a long list of names. "I have a special assignment for you," he tells them. Their body posture suddenly changes. Riccardo recounted, "They say, 'Lord, I'm gonna give this to you for them.' They go from slumped over and 'What's the point of my life?' …to all of a sudden 'I've got work. I've got real work. The Lord needs me' with this new mission and this new meaning."[38]

With this tried-and-true pain management technique, who needs opioids?

If You Give, You Will Receive

The saying "It is better to give than to receive" is a scientifically proven fact. One of the many reasons churchgoers live longer springs from the abundant volunteer opportunities associated with churches. This not only involves donating time and talents to the church itself but also to church-affiliated programs to help the poor, infirm, elderly, youth, imprisoned, and others needing a helping hand. Religious persons volunteer for charitable causes to a much greater extent than the nonreligious, on average. A Gallup poll disclosed that 82 percent of regular churchgoers engage in volunteerism, versus 51 percent for non- or infrequent churchgoers.[39]

Another study concluded churchgoers are more than twice as likely to volunteer to help the needy. Robert Putnam of Harvard and David Campbell of Notre Dame surveyed more than 3,000 people, asking them about religious involvement, civic involvement, and more. They published the findings in their book *American Grace: How Religion Divides and Unites Us*. Churchgoers even volunteer for secular groups nearly twice as much as non-churchgoers. The only area where non-churchgoers volunteer almost as much is arts and cultural organizations. People of faith also are three to four times more likely to be active in their community through membership in leagues, associations, and other groups.[40]

Greater volunteerism among the religious holds true worldwide and across major religions. A Gallup poll conducted in more than 140 countries asked respondents how many times they engaged in certain "helping behaviors" during the past month, confirming that "highly religious" people are more volunteer-oriented than those less so.[41]

Religious teachings are a tremendous incentive for volunteering. Almsgiving and caring for the poor are central tenants of major religions. Christianity teaches that faith without works is dead. (James 2:14-16) Giving to charity, or *Zakat*, is one of the five pillars of Islam. In Judaism, Moses made tithing for the poor an obligation.

In Hinduism and Buddhism, there's *Dāna*, meaning generosity, which can take the form of helping those in need. Inspiration to volunteer also may come from fellow congregants, church leaders, saints in history, or prominent figures in scripture.

Whether it's organized volunteer work or regular informal assistance, the end result is greater wellness. The Corporation for National and Community Service (CNCS) as described in its report *The Health Benefits of Volunteering* reviewed many studies confirming that frequent volunteers have lower rates of mortality and depression. One study uncovered that over a five-year period the mortality rate of elderly who volunteered with two or more organizations was 44 percent lower than non-volunteers. It's mainly the personal sense of accomplishment, meaning and purpose, and self-worth that lead to good outcomes. Just the social interaction that comes with volunteering can engender a mindset of companionship, acceptance, and inclusion, in addition to less loneliness and isolation. And volunteering is more strongly associated with life satisfaction than working for pay.

Eric Kim of the Harvard T.H. Chan School of Public Health and Sara Konrath of the University of Rochester Medical Center observed that volunteers experience more positive emotions, in turn engendering stronger immune systems and improved cardiovascular function. Volunteering's tendency to instill a sense of purpose particularly applies to retired persons who may feel they no longer hold the position in society that they did pre-retirement. It increases the will to live—especially among those who get discouraged easily—prompting them to care more about their health. And since volunteering typically increases the number of people with whom one interacts, it boosts the possibility of seeing or hearing about healthy behaviors.[42]

As further proof that it's better to give than receive, a study of volunteerism among an ethnically diverse array of older adults found that people receiving the support enjoyed no improvement in health. Those providing the support had lower mortality than the non-volunteers.[43]

Volunteering only occasionally—say, an hour a month—doesn't seem to result in better health. To fully reap the benefits you should volunteer about two hours a week over the course of a year. That's a crucial threshold; a study concluded there's little or no health improvement from volunteering less than about a hundred hours per year. Going above and beyond that doesn't appear to result in proportionately greater health benefits.[44] But do it anyway. The world needs your help.

Cornell's Phyllis Moen and colleagues located decades-old interview data on women in upstate New York, and tracked down and re-interviewed 326 of them. It turned out that compared with the less-engaged women, those accustomed to volunteering and participating in clubs or organizations scored higher on functional ability—i.e. ability to carry out everyday activities without health barriers.[45] Volunteering also reduces the risk of cognitive impairment which includes difficulty with memory, speaking, paying attention, and/or recognizing people.[46] And nursing home residents who are given certain responsibilities have greater alertness and well-being than residents who don't have those responsibilities.[47] What about paid work? The Moen study determined that paid caregiving doesn't improve caregivers' health. The explanation offered is that volunteering is more of a discretionary activity with more autonomy, whereas paid work is required of them.[48]

Volunteering is particularly beneficial to people with serious illnesses—to the extent they can volunteer despite those disabilities. It even can yield greater health benefits than medical care itself. When patients with chronic pain began serving as peer volunteers for others undergoing the same kind of suffering, not only did the patient-volunteers' physical pain decrease (yet another alternative to opioids), but they also had lower levels of disability and depression. Another group of heart attack patients who volunteered after their recovery reported reduced despair and depression.

Getting into the habit of volunteering when you're young reduces the risk of health problems later in life, "thereby offering up the possibility that the best way to prevent poor health in the future, which could be a barrier to volunteering, is to volunteer," states CNCS.[49]

Fruits of Faith-Based Volunteerism

Whether the charitable activity is religious or secular, you improve your wellness. But religion-sponsored volunteerism has been found to be more beneficial to health and longevity. Powell and colleagues point out in *American Psychologist* that when helping people in a religious setting, the sense of self-worth in many instances is deeper and broader. The work could be considered to have a sacred quality or be more meaningful because it's done in the context of a higher power.[50] UT Austin's Marc Musick and Duke's John Wilson also contend that volunteering for religious causes is more rewarding and meaningful than nonreligious volunteering, and results in better mental health.[51] Enhanced benefits come from interacting with friends and associates who share similar social and religious worldviews.[52]

UM-Ann Arbor's Neal Krause ascertained that providing informal support and assistance to fellow church members is associated with better health—but only for those deeply committed to their faith. Such support may include providing companionship, transportation, household help, financial assistance, or aiding the sick. This even has greater health benefits than formal volunteer work. Krause suggests it's because informal helpers are more involved with and connected to the people they're benefitting, whereas in the more formal setting they likely aren't deeply involved in the lives of recipients of the aid—and may not even have direct contact with them.[53]

Chapter 3

BELIEF BREEDS HAPPINESS

John grew up without religion. When he was in his early twenties, one day a friend invited him to a church service. Just to be sociable he decided to go. While there, the Holy Spirit came over him and he saw who he was on the inside. He has never looked back. "God, Jesus and the Holy Spirit have changed me from a self-serving unhappy manipulator of other people pursuing an unending and futile search for happiness into a person who considers others in all that I do. As a result I am far happier now than I previously imagined that I ever could be!"[1]

His is one of countless stories of people who found happiness in God. His account echoes that of St. Augustine who observed, "Thou hast made us for Thyself, O Lord, and our heart is restless until it finds its rest in thee."

Edward Diener, professor of psychology (emeritus) at the University of Illinois and co-author along with his son Robert Biswas-Diener of *Happiness: Unlocking the Mysteries of Psychological Wealth*, looked at cultures around the world in an effort to determine what makes people happy. They pinpointed several universal drivers including (in no particular order): supportive relationships, meaningful employment, financial stability, helping others, utilizing one's talents and strengths, being devoted to causes larger than one's self, and religion. It's religion, Diener argues, that helps confer meaning. It can provide a how-to manual for life, with powerful lessons on living ethically, morally, unselfishly, generously, and with less self-centeredness. Religion also:

- enhances people's social networks, enabling befriending of others for support and who share common values and beliefs.

- enables the joy of giving through voluntary or charitable opportunities.

- provides a moral compass through rules of ethical behavior.

- answers large and perplexing questions such as how the universe originated and why evil exists.

- allays fear of death by instilling hope of life after death.

- helps with coping by providing answers to unexplained or uncontrollable events.

The last point was evident in a U.S. study, by Touro College's Steven Pirutinsky and colleagues, of Orthodox Jews' response to the Covid pandemic. Religious devotion and trust in God were associated with a less-negative impact on sleep, diet, family, character, and life satisfaction.[2] In one of his own studies, Diener worked with the Gallup organization to contact a thousand people living in St. Louis through random-digit telephone dialing, enquiring about their life satisfaction. As expected, the ones answering in the affirmative were more likely to believe in God and the afterlife.[3]

Frequency of religious attendance can be a more potent predictor of life satisfaction even than income, education, or health. Lim and Putnam disclosed that 28.2 percent of weekly churchgoers are extremely satisfied, versus 19.6 percent of never-attenders. They write that the difference in life satisfaction between a weekly churchgoer and non-churchgoer is roughly comparable to the difference between someone with "very good" health and another with merely "good" health. And get this: it's also comparable to the difference in life satisfaction between someone with a family income of $100,000 and another of only $10,000.[4] This comports with a study by MIT economists Jonathan Gruber and Sendhil Mullainathan who calculated that going from never attending church to attending weekly is comparable to the effect on happiness of moving from the bottom income quartile to the top quartile.[5] Who needs money to buy happiness when you've got church?

"Religious involvement is related to greater well-being and greater happiness in the vast majority of studies, nearly 80 percent," remarked Koenig. "This is a systematic review. These are not just studies that have been cherry-picked in order to prove a point. This is all of the literature out there that's been published in the English language and is reported in the second edition of the *Handbook of Religion and Health*."[6] Keep in mind that there always will be a handful of studies showing the opposite conclusion. Koenig told a gathering of Army chaplains, "If you study cigarette smoking and its effects on lung cancer, 1 percent will show that it (reduces) lung cancer. I mean that's just the way these studies are. They report different things in different populations. Sometimes they mess up their analyses; they report the opposite of what they actually found. I mean, it's amazing."[7]

If you have toddlers, grade-schoolers or teens, help ensure their happiness now and when they're adults by taking them to church at least once a week. In so doing they have an 18 percent greater likelihood of being happier during their twenties compared with kids who rarely or never go to church, according to Ying Chen and Tyler VanderWeele of Harvard. Get your kids to pray at home frequently as well. That will make them more likely to have higher life satisfaction, be more forgiving, process emotions better, have higher self-esteem, have a greater sense of mission, and be less likely to do drugs or engage in premarital sex.[8] These findings tie in with a study of West Virginia high school students concluding that the more they lived out their religious beliefs, the stronger was their sense of hope, will, purpose, fidelity, love, and care.[9]

Chen and VanderWeele came upon an unexpected finding: daily praying or meditating among adolescents was associated with more rather than fewer physical problems. What accounts for this? They surmised that those with such problems may be more likely to pray in order to cope with their illness. They also suggested people may sometimes avoid medical care, thinking prayer will help them heal.[10]

But physical health problems or not, the data showed that by and large they were happier than the nonreligious.

And degree of happiness, of course, varies from person to person—and country to country. Upon examining the Gallup World Poll, Diener disclosed that in some countries, religious persons reported being less satisfied with their lives than the nonreligious. "It is possible that there are historical or social factors that add to or detract from the potential power of religion in various nations," observed Diener.[11]

The Gallup World Poll poses another paradox. Using data from that poll, the World Happiness Report, published by the United Nations Sustainable Development Solutions Network, lists mainly Scandinavian countries as the happiest.[12] But religiosity in those countries is among the lowest. How to explain? First, it's said there are problems with the methodology.[13] But even if the rankings are correct, recall that religion isn't the only factor influencing happiness. Other factors include income, education, clean environment, freedom, safety and security, and employment. If Scandinavia is happiest, it's for reasons other than religion. Yet, within Scandinavia the happiest people doubtless tend to be the most actively religious. In a news release, Pew Research featured a chart of twenty-six high- and middle-income countries, indicating the percent of each's population who are "very happy" categorized by actively religious, inactively religious, and unaffiliated. In 19 of the 26 countries, the actively religious score highest on "very happy." For the United States, 36 percent of the actively religious are very happy, versus 25 percent for the other two categories.[14] For some reason, Scandinavian countries weren't included in the list.

Another paradox is that countries ranked as happiest in the World Happiness Report tend to rank high in something not so desirable: the incidence of depression and suicide. Curiously, there's no mention of depression or mental illness in the World Happiness Report 2020 (there is in the 2021 report, but only as it relates to Covid-19) and only a passing mention of suicide; one would think these should be factors in compiling its happiness rankings. In any event, we can make an educated guess that in the purportedly happiest countries, the many persons afflicted with depression tend to be the least religious.

It's a similar situation with certain U.S. states including Mississippi and Alabama, which according to surveys have the lowest levels of life satisfaction and overall physical health. Their populations also tend to be the most religious—leading some to erroneously conclude that religion harms health and happiness. But as *Crossroads* points out, among individuals there, the more religious they are, the healthier and happier they tend to be. It's factors other than religion that negatively impact life satisfaction. Jumping to a conclusion based on aggregate or group data while ignoring individual data is known as the "ecological fallacy" in statistics.[15]

The Four Levels of Happiness

Paul was born into a Christian family. Though he didn't often think about God he believed in Him and tried to do the right thing in dealing with others. He worked hard and was considered a success by those who knew him. "Every time I achieved a goal, I expected that achievement to be followed by satisfaction and happiness. I enjoyed the praise and the appearance of success." The happiness never lasted, though. "Inside of my heart and my mind was an emptiness, a hollowness, that 'things,' achievements, and people could not seem to fill." But eventually, circumstances changed. "After I accepted Jesus Christ as my Savior, I came to know what it meant to be satisfied," testified Paul. "I am still a hard worker, but I looked at things from a different perspective. I was no longer empty; I was filled with a sense of purpose that was bigger than the moment. I became hungry to know what the Bible said about being the right kind of husband, the right model of a father, and God's guidelines for business. My outward life may not have changed much, because I had tried to be a moral person. However, on the inside, there was a huge difference. For the first time in my life, I knew contentment."[16]

Happiness is defined as feeling or showing pleasure or contentment. But what kind of contentment, and how deep and long-lasting? In Paul's case, it was genuine—but only after he took on the new attitude. For others, the contentment is ephemeral. Granted, sleeping in or lounging around Sunday morning instead of hoofing it to church could boost short-term happiness. But in making that a habit, would you be happier in the long run? Most likely not.

There's not just one kind of happiness. Father Robert Spitzer, president of the Magis Center for Reason and Faith and former president of Gonzaga University, emphasizes there are four kinds. Levels 1 and 2 are fleeting. True happiness lies with Levels 3 and especially 4—which is where religion comes into play. The four levels are:

Level 1: Immediate Gratification
Level 2: Personal Achievement
Level 3: Contributive
Level 4: Ultimate Good

Level 1 happiness is immediate comfort and pleasure, such as good eats, fun in the sun at the beach, binging on video games, or rocking out to good music. This is fine, but it's only temporary and doesn't run very deep. Many people strive only for this level of happiness, resulting in disappointment or dissatisfaction when the activity ends. Their lives become a constant effort to satisfy short-term gratification.

Level 2 happiness entails ego and self-esteem. It's striving for honor and recognition, whether it be at the workplace, within the community, or anywhere else. Such a goal is valid—up to a point. This type of happiness may last longer than that of Level 1 but it, too, typically is only temporary. For many, Level 2 is the dominant source of happiness; they never get past this level. Sometimes in order to win, others must lose—such as being chosen over someone else for a promotion. Once you achieve that coveted position or distinction, dissatisfaction could set in because there's always something even higher to attain, as happened with Paul. You may even develop suspicions of others thought to be standing in the way of your rise. "If my life gets stuck in Level 2 as my dominant source of happiness, I will be constantly obsessed with seeking that next win, and paranoid that others are trying to keep me from it," relates Spitzer.[17]

Level 3 happiness is deeper and more enduring. It focuses on serving others rather than one's self. This may involve donating generously to charitable causes, volunteering your time for charity or to help the community, or accepting a job with lower pay than what you otherwise could earn in order to be part of a worthy cause. You achieve happiness knowing you're positively impacting others.

To be sure, it can be easy for Level 2 happiness to creep in, such as donating a lot of money or time in order to be publicly recognized. You could enjoy aspects of Level 3 happiness but ultimately be stuck at Level 2. "Be careful not to parade your uprightness in public to attract attention; otherwise you will lose all reward from your Father in heaven," admonished Jesus. (Matthew 6:1) Granted, sometimes you can't avoid being recognized. If that happens, don't let it go to your head.

Level 4 is the deepest and most solid type of happiness. It involves yearning for or achieving truth, goodness, love, beauty, and being, and not through the material things of the world. Those achieving Level 4 happiness may not even care about Levels 1 and 2. Many saints, for example, lived lives of poverty and humility yet were quite happy serving God and others. True happiness is found through the spiritual and transcendent—i.e. through God.[18] "God cannot give us a happiness and peace apart from Himself," writes the renowned British writer and theologian C.S. Lewis. He explains that just as a (gas-powered) car is designed to run only on gasoline and would sputter and stall on anything else, God designed humans to run only on Himself. "It is just no good asking God to make us happy in our own way without bothering about religion."[19]

Levels 1 and 2 happiness is summed up in these seven P's—pleasure, possessions, praise, prestige, popularity, power, and position.[20]

But those alone usually fall short. Vis-à-vis Level 3, religions commonly teach that aiding others not only is righteous for its own sake but also necessary for salvation. Level 4 stems from having a strong sense of meaning and purpose, especially knowing we're deeply loved by our eternal Creator.

> "Not one (sparrow) falls to the ground without your Father's knowledge. Even all the hairs of your head are counted. So do not be afraid; you are worth more than many sparrows." (Matthew 10:29-31)

Christianity conveys that the present world is but a shadow of the eternal world. Living by God's teachings as laid out in the Bible positions us for that world. The Christian meaning of life is commonly summed up with the words of St. Ignatius of Loyola: To know, love, and serve God in this world so we can be happy with Him in the next.

Most religions have an explanation for how the world arose, and for what purpose. Christianity teaches that in the beginning there was God. He created a high-tier life form endowed with free will, the angels. Many of them rebelled and became fallen angels, embodying evil. God created a lower-tier life form, humans, also possessing free will. Lower still are animals and other life forms. Humans rebelled early on, displeasing God and giving rights to the fallen angels to roam the world and wreak havoc among us humans—helping to explain why there's evil in the world. God instituted a plan of salvation, culminating with God himself entering the world in human form, and sacrificing himself to atone for the sins of humankind. Those who embrace this paradigm find tremendous comfort and meaning in it.

An atheist, by contrast, typically believes the world and its inhabitants arose through chance and accident, with no ultimate meaning. This can generate considerable angst—as apparently happened to Jesse Kilgore. After the college student read Richard Dawkins' *The God Delusion* he lost his faith along with a sense of meaning and purpose, according to his friends. Tragically, he committed suicide (although other preexisting issues may have prompted it).[21] To be sure, many atheists would argue that one can find meaning and purpose in ways other than religion. And Kilgore may have been fine with the thought of nonexistence after death. But for many it's a horrifying thought. It's much more comforting to believe there's an afterlife—especially a blissful one—than to believe your consciousness vanishes when your brain stops working. As Koenig observes, "Religious beliefs provide satisfying answers to existential questions, such as 'where did we come from', 'why are we here', and 'where are we going', and the answers apply to both this life and the next life, thus reducing existential angst."[22] That's another reason why people of faith are happier. And it extends to the very end of life. Terminally ill patients who believe in the afterlife have lower levels of despair compared with those who don't believe.[23] They have plenty of backup in the abundant peer-reviewed academic studies on near-death experiences showing that consciousness lives on after clinical death.[24]

"Hope is really important—that things have a purpose, that God can take something bad and turn it around into something good… and knowing that there's life after death," remarked Koenig in an interview with Dr. Laurie Marbas. He said that for a materialist (one who believes that nothing beyond the material world exists), "The outlook there is pretty dim…There's no purpose or meaning to this life and when we die that's it, there's no resting in peace. There's non-existence for all of eternity. But religion says, 'No, there are other sources of truths, and we don't understand everything right now, and there just might be something more to this life.'"[25]

That must partly explain why as a profession, the happiest and most satisfied of all Americans are clergy members.[26] Catholic University of America's Stephen Rossetti ran a statistical analysis to pin down the strongest factor behind Catholic priests' happiness. It's inner peace. As further confirmation of St. Augustine's dictum that "Our heart is restless until it finds its rest in thee," Rossetti crunched the numbers to ascertain that the most important predictor of inner peace is a strong relationship with God.[27] Clergy also are more heart-healthy; a study disclosed that compared with the general population, Baptist ministers are 40 percent less likely to die from heart disease.[28]

Many things boost Level 1 or 2 happiness that all too often lead to long-term angst. They include drinking, drugs, pornography, extramarital sex, gambling, and obsession with status and with status symbols, to name a few. Still other activities can both boost short-term happiness and engender long-term happiness, such as listening to inspiring music. Or they may have a neutral or even negative effect on short-term happiness, such as getting up early for church, but result in long-term happiness. Religion quite often spawns not just an ephemeral happiness but a deep and abiding one.

As with John discussed at the beginning of this chapter, stories of people finding God and turning their life around are legion. Another case in point is Michelle:

"I was suffering from a terrible depression that led me to start thinking about suicide. Around that time I was talking to some people on a few forums about my problems. One of those people helped me learn a little bit about Jesus. I also found out about prayer on the Internet, which led me to read about Jesus. Eventually, I began to realize that even the person who had helped me learn some about Jesus, couldn't help me. It seemed like the only one who could help me was the Lord himself. I felt like I couldn't trust people, so I turned to the Lord. Now I'm doing a lot better and I'm no longer suicidal. I trust people more and the Lord has changed me so much! Thanks to Jesus, I no longer want to die! If it wasn't for him I do not think I would have made it. That's not all he's done though; He has saved me so I could have everlasting life!"[29]

Mind you, churchgoing and faith in God don't guarantee happiness. In Christianity, earthly happiness is by no means the main goal. Jesus never promised it. In fact, he warned that Christians will have their share of hardship, suffering, temptation, and tribulation—such as when following the teachings of Jesus rather than the teachings of the secular world, when the two conflict. But whatever hardships Christians go through are different in degree and kind from the hardships people endure when living a life far from the laws of God. With the latter, the difficulties are usually worse. (Things could get considerably worse after they depart this world.)

Stressing the Positive

Less stress usually means greater happiness. A study published in *Psychological Science* revealed that thinking about God or religion can reduce the stress or anxiety associated with making mistakes. The researchers had study participants write about religion or do a word scramble that included religion and God-related words. Then they carried out a computerized task programmed to result in a high rate of errors in an effort to elicit a distress-response, which was quantified based on measuring brain waves. The investigators monitored the anterior cingulate cortex (ACC), which serves an alerting function when wrong outcomes occur. Sure enough, amid the test errors, the group prepped with religious thoughts had lower activity in the ACC, i.e. a lower level of distress, than the group without such prepping. The results held true whether the religious thoughts were conscious or unconscious.

The experiments showed that contemplating religion and God mitigates anxiety associated with making mistakes and helps people take setbacks in stride. "Thinking about religion makes you calm under fire. It makes you less distressed when you've made an error," Michael Inzlicht told *LiveScience*.[30] Inzlicht coauthored the study with Alexa Tullett, both of the University of Toronto Scarborough. In their paper they observed, "More broadly, our results may offer a mechanism for the finding that religion is linked to positive mental health and low rates of mortality and morbidity. If thinking about religion leads people to react to their errors with less distress and defensiveness—an effect that occurs within a few hundredths of a second—in the long run, this effect may translate to religious people living their life with greater equanimity than nonreligious people, being better able to cope with the pressures of living in a sometimes hostile world." (Interestingly, when atheists were unconsciously presented with God-related impressions, their ACC activity increased—i.e. greater distress. This suggests they're so committed to the notion of no God that anything contradicting that causes some anxiety. But don't give up on them—they may come around sooner or later.)[31]

The Middle East is where things really can get hostile. Israeli researchers measured stress levels of devout Jews living in the Gaza Strip where the threat of violent attacks was omnipresent. Compared with two other groups of Israelis living in equally violence-prone areas and who generally were secular-minded, the Gaza Strip Jews had less stress and the lowest sense of personal threat. Wrote the study authors, "Deeply held belief systems affecting life-views may impart significant resilience to developing stress-related problems, even under extreme conditions."[32]

Trust and Gratitude

One of the most often-cited reasons people give in explaining their happiness is their faith. The highly religious are more likely to be "very happy with the way things are going in life," according to a Pew poll.[33] Of 99 studies that Objective Hope reviewed on this subject, 79 found a positive association between religious involvement and greater happiness, life satisfaction, morale, positive affectivity (a fancy term psychologists use to describe enthusiasm, happiness, and other positive emotions), or some other measure of well-being. Eleven found no association and eight came up with mixed results. Only one study found a negative association, which involved a small and nonrandom sample of college students.[34] In Koenig's systematic review, 82 percent of studies with the highest methodological rigor had a positive association, and only one was negative.[35]

Religion also boosts self-esteem. But this isn't based on worldly characteristics, in which self-esteem is derived from physical appearance, individual accomplishments, material possessions, educational attainment, level of respect from peers, and the like. Self-esteem should depend on your spiritual state—what God thinks of you, not what people think of you. Of the 24 studies that Objective Hope reviewed on religious commitment and self-esteem, 15 found a positive association, six no association, two mixed, and only one negative.

One of those studies found that regular churchgoers have a lot more "faith in people" compared with infrequent or non-attenders.

Churchgoing adolescents tended to agree with the statements, "Most people are more inclined to help others than to look out for themselves," and "Human nature is fundamentally cooperative." Non-churchgoers by contrast tended to agree with: "Most people cannot be trusted; you can't be too careful in your dealings with people," "If you don't watch yourself, people will take advantage of you," and "The lot of the average person is getting worse."[36]

More trusting people are happier. They also typically have a keener sense of gratitude—towards others and/or God. Gratitude has been shown to foster a sense of meaning, social bonds and friendships, optimism, progress toward personal goals, altruism, and a greater sense of social responsibility. It's even associated with exercise, better health, and better sleep quality. The more you pray, the greater your sense of gratitude, reveal Florida State's Nathaniel Lambert and colleagues in their study "Can Prayer Increase Gratitude?" A daily prayer ritual often includes counting one's blessings. Praying leads to being grateful to God for things normally taken for granted such as the beauty of nature, the air you breathe, and life in general. "Gratitude is a burgeoning topic of research and shows promise as a mechanism for enhancing physical and mental health. Prayer is a widespread religious practice that is gaining momentum as a potential tool for clinicians—where culturally appropriate," writes the study team.[37]

Harold Koenig affirmed that religion-inspired gratitude and forgiveness can make a real difference in a person's health, and said there's a lot of research backing that up. "Being thankful for what one has rather than focusing and obsessing on what one does not have can affect a person's mental health in many ways, particularly with regard to generating positive emotions such as well-being, life satisfaction, a sense of happiness, and fullness of life. When a person is grateful and is forgiving others, those emotions just kind of bubble up from deep inside," remarked Koenig. And of course, the mental affects the physical. Ungrateful and/or unforgiving persons are prone to weaker immune systems and susceptibility to infection, particularly during times of pandemic. "So not only does religious faith, gratitude, and forgiveness enhance a person's mental health and well-being, it enhances their physical health and longevity," he affirmed.[38]

The Hell Factor

Does the notion of eternal damnation affect happiness? Diener found that believers in hell and the devil are slightly less happy than those who only believe in heaven[39] (but presumably happier than their atheist or agnostic counterparts). This is understandable; pondering the reality of hell and Jesus's numerous references to it in the Gospels are enough to cause distress—just as the prospect of prison could generate some anxiety in a criminal or potential criminal. Books such as *The Dogma of Hell* by Rev. F.X. Schouppe and *The Four Last Things* by Fr. Martin Von Cochem give frightening depictions of hell, in part based on supernatural visions of saints and other mystics. Personal testimonies of near-death or out-of-body experiences involving alleged visits to hell—abundantly available on YouTube and elsewhere—can be distressing to watch as well. It can stem from worry over the possibility of ending up in hell oneself, and/or one's nonreligious relatives and friends suffering that fate.

Diener's conclusion introduces a paradox. Typically, the more religiously devout the person, the happier he or she is. On the other hand, the more religiously devout, the more strongly he or she tends to believe in hell and the devil (in addition to heaven). Those who only believe in heaven are less prone to attend church or to pray, partly based on the line of reasoning that if everyone is guaranteed heaven, why bother with church? Yet it's those people who are inclined to be less happy.

Diener also writes that members of religions that claim theirs is the only way to salvation tend to have lower life satisfaction.[40] This is another curious finding. In Christianity, Jesus exclaims, "I am the way, the truth, and the life. No one comes to the Father except through me." (John 14:6) This implies Christianity is the only way to salvation. But do serious Christians have lower life satisfaction? In general, no.

Natural and Supernatural Pathways

In sum, religion boosts happiness through the following natural mechanisms or "active ingredients": certain beliefs and attitudes including having a strong sense of meaning and purpose; social support and interaction; and focusing on others and God rather than on self.

The believer takes comfort in knowing he or she is made in God's image and likeness, and that God can make something good out of every situation as long as trust is placed in Him. He's available anytime and anywhere through prayer, to offer strength and hope.[41] He's not just a God of justice but also of mercy, ready to forgive past sins so long as there's repentance and renewal. Other happiness-generating attitudes include forgiveness, gratitude, generosity, kindness, and believing each of us is here for a God-designed purpose.

Religion also brings people together for worship, learning, discussion, service projects, casual chat, and celebrations. Social connectedness is an instinctive need; absence thereof leads to abnormal brain activity. The chemistry and biology of how social interaction boosts our mental health are as yet largely unknown, according to Harvard researchers.[42] However, theories have been put forth. For example, our hearts produce electromagnetic energy fields which may interact when we're in proximity to other people, with salutary effects.[43]

Loving thy neighbor as thyself (Matthew 22:39) is another conduit toward happiness, in which self-sacrifice and the (largely unremunerated) serving of others carry the day. "It's also a higher quality of support," said Koenig. "Religious people do it partly for the social exchange, but they have an additional motivation that others don't. And that is to love your neighbor as yourself. Even if it's hard, even if they give you nothing back, you are to unconditionally love your neighbor."[44]

Those are natural pathways of how religion leads to happiness. There's also a supernatural pathway: direct graces from God. More on that in chapter 13.

Chapter 4

DEFEATING DEPRESSION, DRUGS, AND DRINK

The famed Swiss psychiatrist Carl Jung observed, "Among all my patients in the second half of life—that is to say, over thirty-five—there has not been one whose problem in the last resort was not that of finding a religious outlook on life. It is safe to say that every one of them fell ill because he had lost that which the living religions of every age have given their followers, and none of them has been really healed who did not regain his religious outlook."[1] That's strong testimony to the power of faith in staving off depression.

It's no coincidence that mental illnesses are at all-time highs while churchgoing and belief in God are at all-time lows. In any given year about 1 in 5 U.S. adults (or 1 in 4 depending on the statistics used) suffers from a diagnosable mental disorder.[2] The problem is most acute in younger people, among whom religious belief and practice are declining fastest. From 2009 through 2019, eighteen- to twenty-five year-olds who had suffered a mental illness within the past year went from 18.0 percent to 29.4 percent of that population. That's an astonishing 63 percent increase in only a decade. Those experiencing "major depressive episode with severe impairment" doubled from 5.2 percent to 10.3 percent of that age group, and from 5.8 percent to 11.1 percent among twelve- to seventeen-year-olds.[3]

All that was pre-Covid. The social isolation during that pandemic resulted in intentional-self harm among teenagers skyrocketing 100 percent at the beginning of the lockdowns compared with the year-prior period. Depression, overdoses, substance abuse, obsessive-compulsive disorders, and tic disorders were up by similar amounts.[4]

Of course, multiple factors are behind the rise in mental illness. In addition to social isolation, they include the proliferation of electronic communication and digital media, particularly via smartphones, which discourage face-to-face interaction. Other factors include the rise of opioids and fewer hours of sleep.[5] But a prominent factor is the decline in religious practice. In 1999, 70 percent of Americans said they belonged to a church, synagogue, or mosque. In 2020 that had plummeted to 47 percent.[6] And from 2009 through 2019:[7]

- The percentage of U.S. adults unaffiliated with any religion shot up from 17 to 26 percent.

- Among those born between 1981 and 1996, the unaffiliated climbed from 27 to 40 percent of that age group.

- The frequency of those going to church at least once a week plummeted from 47 percent of U.S. adults to 40 percent.

- Those reporting never going to church rose from 13 percent to 19 percent.

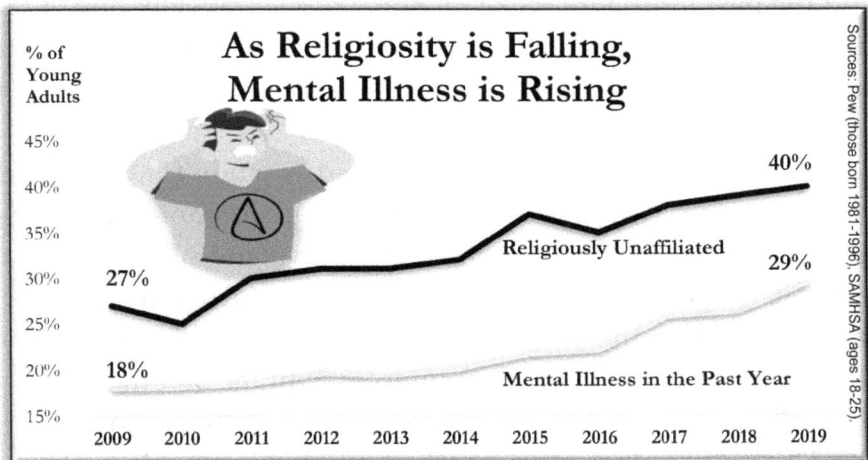

As Religiosity is Falling, Mental Illness is Rising

% of Young Adults

45%
40%
35%
30%
25%
20%
15%

27%
18%

40%

Religiously Unaffiliated

29%

Mental Illness in the Past Year

2009 2010 2011 2012 2013 2014 2015 2016 2017 2018 2019

Sources: Pew (those born 1981-1996), SAMHSA (ages 18-25)

Best Medicine for the Blues

With such huge and growing numbers of people without faith, the plagues of depression and other forms of mental illness will worsen. If you're at risk for depression or anxiety and don't have a church community, find one. Pray and read sacred scripture often. As it says in the Bible, "Have no anxiety about anything, but in everything by prayer and supplication with thanksgiving let your requests be made known to God." (Philippians 4:6) If you harbor doubts about the existence of a loving and caring God, see the last chapter for starters.

Aleaya had her doubts. But she prayed anyway. During her freshman year of high school she descended into anxiety and depression. It got so bad that one day in the shower she started bawling her eyes out. "This was the first point in my life where I felt like I had nothing else to live for." She remembers lying in bed and looking up at the ceiling. "And I was like, I'm going to pray about this. And I hate praying in these situations because I always feel so awkward. I'm like, God is probably judging me or laughing at me, like this is so dumb...But in this situation I decided to pray about it...I just felt so much better. I just remember feeling like I was going to be okay and it was tripping my mind out because just a few seconds earlier I was wanting to die over this problem...I fell right to sleep and the next morning I woke up and I was completely fine. It felt like nothing had happened...I seriously decided to give my life to Jesus and actually get saved...I was able to just pray and ask him into my life and he's been there ever since."[8]

When you're sad, angry, or distressed, wouldn't it be great to have a loving, caring and understanding companion available anytime and anywhere? That's what Aleaya and so many others enjoy. They perceive God as providing powerful support whether or not it's during times of trouble. "To be able to just sit down and think that God wanted to communicate with me and that I'm not a scumbag in front of His eyes no matter what. Wow, how cool is that?," said a Southern Baptist who had an abusive husband.[9]

Active worship is associated with less anger, hostility, and aggressiveness. It tends to mitigate stress by calming, promoting meaningful social relationships, and reducing bad habits.[10] It provides a framework for the world and explains seemingly random and problematic events.[11] Monthly churchgoing lowers the odds of depression, but not by as much as doing so weekly.[12] Of the 103 studies *Objective Hope* reviewed on the religion-depression relationship, 70 of them found less depression, 17 no association, 12 mixed results, and only 4 found a negative effect.[13] Of the 178 studies with the highest methodological rigor in Koenig's systematic review, 119 were associated with less depression and just 13 with more.[14]

At the Islamic Azad University of Ahvaz, Iran, researchers surveyed 300 Muslim students, finding significantly fewer mental disorders among the more religious ones. "Behaviors such as trust in God, prayer, pilgrimage...can lead to inner calm through hope and encouragement to positive attitudes," write the investigators.[15] In a systematic review of the research on mental health among Muslims, Koenig along with Saad Saleh Al Shohaib of King Abdulaziz University also found a positive relationship. It's largely based on strong faith, frequent prayer, recitation of the Koran and careful adherence to its teachings, and a supportive and cohesive family and Muslim community.[16]

The previous chapter highlights Level 3 happiness—brought about by focusing on others rather than self. Nonreligious people engage in charitable activities all the time, and it no doubt alleviates depression and makes them happier. But they're missing out on something even better: church. Chapter 1 points to the London School of Economics and Erasmus University study finding that secular social engagement isn't nearly as effective in stomping out depression as religious-oriented engagement. Commenting on the study, *Time* writer Brian Walsh wrote, "It's as if a sense of spirituality and an active, social religious practice were an effective vaccine against the virus of unhappiness."[17]

The stronger your faith, the faster your recovery from depression. Koenig tracked eighty-seven physically ill patients at Duke University Hospital, following up with them every three months after discharge. He gauged their intrinsic religiosity, defined as those whose "master motive" is religion—who put their faith above all else. Without prompting, when asked how they cope with their physical illness, such patients answered "my faith," "prayer," "the Lord," "Jesus," "God," and the like. They were given a questionnaire measuring religiosity. For every ten-point increase in intrinsic religiosity, recovery from depression was 70 percent faster after discharge. For those whose physical conditions worsened or failed to improve, it was 100 percent faster.[18] What fuels the faster recovery? Koenig suggested strong religious belief provides a worldview that enables acceptance of physical illness, pain, suffering, and death. It engenders a self-esteem that's more robust than a self-esteem based on worldly matters such as material goods and physical qualities.[19]

That's ironic, because so many people disbelieve in God because they can't imagine He ever would allow suffering. One reason He allows it is that it so often prompts people to turn toward Him. The Covid pandemic bears this out. In a Pew poll, 24 percent of the respondents' faith had become stronger because of the pandemic, and for only 2 percent it was weaker—despite the wave of church closures.[20] And stronger faith makes them better able to cope. A Brazilian study revealed that during Covid lockdowns, more frequent praying and other religious activities were associated with lower levels of worrying, fear, and sadness.[21] Another study reported that those whose religiosity declined during Covid were twice as likely to feel isolated and lonely.[22]

Religion helps focus your mind on things beyond rather than the pain and suffering of the earth. "Worshiping together with the religious congregation may offer the disabled elderly person a route, through prayer, or receiving the sacraments, or appreciation of the beauty of the place, to a transcendent state in which the body and its frailties don't matter much," write Idler and Kasl. "The motivation to return to this state, and to the accompanying social support and pleasant pastimes that religious groups provide, may be a strong factor influencing the recovery of elderly people with new disabilities."[23]

To cope with the burdens of life and break free of depression or prevent a descent into it, individuals often invoke thoughts of the benevolence of God and seek to connect with Him. They may solicit support from clergy and other church members, or even provide spiritual guidance to others.[24] Of course, there are plenty of nonreligious coping strategies as well. But the religious kind are as good if not better. "Associations between religious coping behaviors and mental health status are at least as strong, if not stronger, than those observed with nonreligious coping behaviors," write Koenig and colleagues. They conducted a study of 577 depressed patients, examining various types of religious coping methods. Included are negative religious coping methods. Such persons may express anger at God for unfortunate events, feel God is punishing them for sins or lack of spirituality, or may hope God punishes others for the same. Much of this is sinful behavior contrary to biblical teachings, and not surprisingly, is associated with worse mental and physical health. These people may have a less-secure relationship with God and an ominous and foreboding view of the world, amid a sometimes-futile search for purpose and meaning in their lives.[25]

Far more common are positive religious coping methods. One such method is ritualistic prayer. Matthew Anastasi and Andrew Newberg of UPenn sought to determine the effects of ritualistic prayer on anxiety, choosing the Rosary as their medium of study. They had a group of Catholic participants pray the Rosary and another group watch a religious-themed video for a half-hour, measuring their level of anxiety before and after. As a whole, the video group experienced no significant decrease in anxiety, but the Rosary group did. While pointing out that high religiosity is associated with better health in the long run, the study authors wrote that in the short run, various studies have shown that "meditative rituals decrease anxiety and depression as well as lower blood-lactate levels and blood pressure." Other studies have confirmed the anxiety-lessening effects of the Rosary, and have shown that God-centered meditation reduces anxiety more than secular med-itation and relaxation exercises.[26]

Newberg, author of *Neurotheology: How Science Can Enlighten Us About Spirituality*, has studied meditation and religious experience extensively, scanning the brains of Catholic nuns, Buddhist monks, chanting Sikhs, and many others in an effort to assess the benefits of prayer and meditation. (Note that the latter is often associated with Eastern religions, but there's Christian and Jewish meditation as well.) His research shows that these practices change the brain over time, particularly the frontal lobe and thalamus. "The brain changes reported to be associated with religious and spiritual prac-tices hint at how they also reduce anxiety and depression while enhancing compassion and love," he wrote.[27] In one study, Newberg instructed older people with memory problems to practice daily meditation. After eight weeks, many of them reported a substantial improvement in memory in addition to being better able to focus and think clearly.[28]

The cerebral cortex is the thick, highly folded outer portion of the brain, comprising about half its weight. Thinning of the cerebral cortex is associated with various neurodegenerative and psychiatric disorders. Using magnetic resonance imaging on a study sample of 103 adults, a Columbia University team who published their find-ings in *JAMA Psychiatry* determined that people who consider their faith life to be highly important have thicker cortices compared with those for whom religion is of low or moderate importance. Blood flow to the affected regions is higher among the more religious, including those who meditate. The difference in cortical thickness particularly stands out for persons at high risk for depression based on family history. In an earlier study the same researchers found that holding religion in high importance decreases the high-risk group's likelihood of depression by 90 percent. (To see brain scans juxtaposing religious and non-religious persons, refer to the study "Neuroanatomical Correlates of Religiosity and Spirituality: A Study in Adults at High and Low Familial Risk for Depression.")

What about someone who regularly attends church yet doesn't consider religion to be highly important—i.e. what's known as extrinsic religiosity? This isn't associated with cortical thickness.[29] So don't just be a pew warmer.

As with adults, churchgoing teenagers with high spirituality enjoy lower rates of depression than non-churchgoing teens who don't put religion at front and center. A team of Southwest Texas State professors ranked levels of depression according to frequency of churchgoing and spirituality, based on the Beck Depression Inventory. Developed by the prominent psychiatrist Aaron T. Beck, it's a twenty-one-question multiple-choice survey widely used for measuring intensity of depression. Teens classified as high in spirituality answered yes to the following questions: "Religion is especially important to me because it answers many questions about the meaning of my life," and "I try hard to carry my religion into my other dealings in life because my religious beliefs are what really lie behind my whole approach to life." Following are the results:[30]

Teen boys - happiest/least depressed to least happy/most depressed:

Frequent churchgoing with high spirituality
Frequent churchgoing with low spirituality
Infrequent churchgoing with high spirituality
Infrequent churchgoing with low spirituality

Teen girls - happiest/least depressed to least happy/most depressed:

Frequent churchgoing with high spirituality
Infrequent churchgoing with high spirituality
Frequent churchgoing with low spirituality
Infrequent churchgoing with low spirituality

Go All Out

To avoid depression, go full bore—be very religious rather than moderately so. Across religions, the more religiously orthodox the

person—i.e. carefully following all precepts of the faith—the greater the likelihood of good mental health.[31] This is borne out in the
Gallup-Healthways Well-Being Index showing that very religious
persons are 17 percent less likely to be diagnosed with depression
during their lifetime than nonreligious. And interestingly, according to the same survey the very religious are 24 percent less likely
to have had depression than the moderately religious. If this is
accurate, it tells us that moderately religious persons are more
likely to be depressed than nonreligious. Why? There's a "complex
pattern of the interplay of religion and emotional wellbeing among
those who are not at the top end of the religious scale," according
to the Gallup analysts. It's a "non-linear relationship between religiosity and emotional well-being," i.e. from the lowest level of religiosity to the highest, the level of psychological benefit isn't necessarily a steady increase. There may be ups and downs along the
way—but ultimately it goes up.[32]

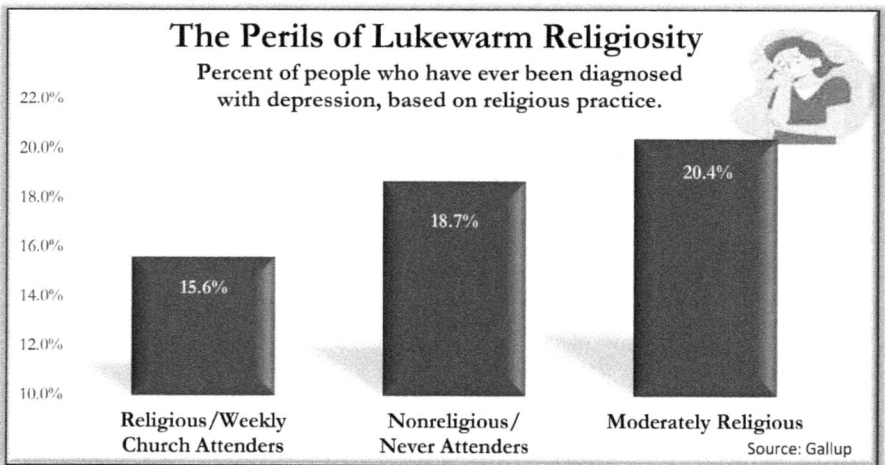

The Perils of Lukewarm Religiosity
Percent of people who have ever been diagnosed
with depression, based on religious practice.

Religious/Weekly Church Attenders	Nonreligious/Never Attenders	Moderately Religious
15.6%	18.7%	20.4%

Source: Gallup

This certainly does not necessarily mean an atheist or agnostic
who decides to embrace church will initially be less happy and only
become happier as his or her faith grows. The non-linear relationship applies more to disparate groups of persons, each at various
levels of religiosity, many of whom are stuck there. Someone's heart
may not be into their faith, perhaps because they were never prop-

erly catechized or because they let the affairs of the world drown out the affairs of God. It's this person, who has no plans to embrace their faith or grow in it, who's more susceptible to depression.

There's a risk depressed churchgoers will stop attending. That, in turn, exacerbates their woes. VanderWeele recommends that religious leaders be cognizant of those with depression and offer support and possible referral before it worsens. It's also possible that negative interactions among fellow church members could lead to distress.[33]

The last point brings up an interesting irony: it's part of being human that social interaction will sometimes involve misunderstandings, disputes, personality conflicts, jealousies, resentments, arguments, and tussles (yes, even at church), all of which can bring on distress. Yet, it's scientifically confirmed that social interaction is associated with greater happiness and health. So when dealing with people in general, the good outweighs the bad.

Meanwhile, churchgoing's tendency to alleviate depression seems greater for women than for men, reports VanderWeele. However, another study found that church could be a source of stress for unmarried teen mothers, likely because of religious teachings against nonmarital sexual relations.[34] According to Christian principles, based on the story of the adulteress about to be stoned (John 8:1-11), such unmarried mothers should be welcomed and forgiven, but gently advised to limit sexual relations only to marriage.

Finally, unless you happen to get filled with the Holy Spirit in a bout of religious ecstasy, don't have the attitude that a few church services will instantly cure you. It takes time and commitment.

Beating Booze and Drugs

In Mexico, heavy drinkers take pledges to stay sober. But it's not just any pledge, like a new year's resolution. It's a pledge to the mother of Jesus Christ, the Blessed Virgin Mary. Before an image or statue of her in the form of the Virgin of Guadalupe (the patron saint of Mexico) and in the presence of a Catholic priest, they promise not to drink for a set period of time. This is known as a *Juramento*, translated as "oath." In addition to no drinking or drugs, the pledger may do penance and offer prayers.

Every so often, Mr. Sanchez takes such an oath. When his friends pressure him into having a drink, he shows them his *Juramento* "ticket" from the church. They understand and respect it. While he may resume drinking at a later date, *Juramentos* are effective in getting him to cut down. When his binges get unbearable for his wife, she threatens to leave him unless he makes another pledge to the Blessed Virgin. He does so, and is sober for weeks or months. He starts drinking again, and she tolerates it until she again tells him she's leaving, and the cycle repeats. Though he returns to drinking, each time he typically lengthens the abstinence.

Mr. Sanchez told his story to Mary Cuadrado and Louis Lieberman of UT El Paso who researched *Juramentos* among Mexican immigrants. The scholars observe that it reinforces willpower and helps appease friends and loved ones concerned about the person's drinking. Others are happy to help him on a *Juramento*. "The cycle of relapse and increased length of abstinence is one that is often recognized by U.S. treatment providers (including AA) as an expected stage that may eventually lead to total abstinence," write Cuadrado and Lieberman. It also "may provide a culturally sensitive adjunct for treatment of Mexican and other Hispanic clients in the United States."[35]

The faith angle is such a powerful weapon against alcohol abuse that it hasn't escaped the notice of Alcoholics Anonymous—to the extent that AA is commonly erroneously thought to be affiliated with a religious organization. Standard fare at AA meetings are the Our Father and the Serenity Prayer. In its vaunted 12-step program, seven of the steps refer to God, a higher power, or the spiritual. (Many atheists and agnostics weren't comfortable with the religious overtones, prompting AA to start support groups catering to them.)[36] Other 12-step programs integrating religion are Porn Anonymous, Gamblers Anonymous, and Chronic Pain Anonymous.

Alcohol and drug abuse are on the upswing. An estimated 25 percent of adult Americans binge drink (6 percent of adults are heavy drinkers). Almost 20 percent of those twelve or older used illegal drugs or misused prescription drugs within the year prior to being surveyed. Drug overdose deaths skyrocketed from 6.9 per 100,000 in 1999 to 22.7 per 100,000 in 2019, a 230 percent increase. Alcohol-induced deaths increased by 70 percent during that time.[37]

Tara got sucked into that trap. At age sixteen she was heavily into drugs and alcohol. Eight years later the situation still was the same. "One day, I felt I had hit rock bottom and needed help. I cried out to the Lord, and He was there for me. Eventually, He freed me from all drugs. I have been clean for six years, praise God. I know I couldn't have quit on my own, but the Lord took it all away from me. Now I have three beautiful children that know the Lord, and a husband that is learning. I still have a struggle with alcohol, but the Lord is doing a work in me. He has saved me so many times from the grip of hell, I know He will do it again."[38]

Tara's story shows that in confronting the scourge of substance abuse, church institutions are crucial. The more religious a person or family is, the less likely abuse will occur.[39] Objective Hope reviewed more than 150 studies examining the relationship between drug and alcohol abuse, and religiosity. The vast majority—87 percent and 94 percent of the drug and alcohol studies respectively—ascertained that regardless of the type of group studied (e.g. adolescents or adults), greater religiosity is associated with less abuse. Koenig's systematic review had similar results.[40]

As reported by Patrick Fagan of the Marriage and Religion Research Institute, alcohol abuse among church avoiders is an astounding 300 percent higher than among churchgoers.[41] A study published in the *Journal of Religion and Health* found that churchgoing middle- and high school students in the Dominican Republic displayed less alcohol consumption than their non-churchgoing peers, fewer intoxications, and a higher age at which they took their first drink.[42] It's a similar story with drugs; nonreligious and especially non-churchgoing people are more likely to abuse them. Addicts tend to pray and read the Bible far less, and frequently stopped attending church during adolescence. In the U.S., religious youth from low-income neighborhoods are not only less likely to use illegal drugs compared with nonreligious youth around them, but also compared with nonreligious youth in higher-income neighborhoods. And just to be religious isn't enough; it's regular church attendance that's associated with less drug use. Moreover, churchgoers who've abused drugs and alcohol are more likely than the nonreligious to recover from such struggles. The more religious the alcoholic, the more likely he or she is to seek treatment, according to Fagan.[43]

A denomination doesn't even have to teach against the use and abuse of alcohol, and still, it's lower within that denomination. To be sure, drug and alcohol avoidance is highest within those that do forbid their use, such as the Mormon faith. The most conservative religious denominations show the lowest drug and alcohol use. A study found that alcohol use is highest among Catholics and Jews.[44] The Catholic Church teaches against drunkenness, but not against consuming in moderation. It's obvious that too many Catholics have a loose definition of moderation.

Drugs, drink, and depression are amounting to untold numbers of what are known as deaths of despair. Fueling the rise are the plummeting number of people in pews Sunday mornings. Women who attend weekly church services have a 68 percent lower risk of death from despair compared with non-churchgoers. For men it's a 33 percent lower risk. Technically that's among health care professionals, on whom surveys were done. But Ying Chen and her Harvard colleagues who calculated these risks indicate that the results are important in understanding factors behind deaths of despair in the population as a whole.[45]

Chapter 5

CHURCH CULTIVATES INTEGRITY AND SELF-DISCIPLINE

"The notion that God is watching you even when others are not is probably the most powerful civilizing force in all of human history." So writes author and commentator Jonah Goldberg.[1] He's right. The perception that a higher being or beings are watching your every move, and that punishment in the afterlife awaits misbehavers, is potent incentive to live ethically and charitably. That, in turn, benefits mind, body, and community.

In civil society, would-be troublemakers fear jail, fines, lawsuits, loss of job, loss of friends, or tarnished reputation. Bolstering those deterrents are robust enforcement mechanisms such as strong police presence, video surveillance, paper trails, and electronic footprints. Surveillance cameras not only help catch criminals but deter crime; when people know they're being observed, they tend to behave (albeit certainly not always, as any reality show will attest).

But when laws are weak and/or when enforcement breaks down, people shirk the rules and do things that can harm others, such as speeding, drunk driving, bribery, theft, or assault. And there are plenty of ways to act unethically even while not breaking the law. This includes lying, back-stabbing, deceit, selfishness, cheating, prejudice, slander, infidelity, perversion, alcohol abuse, cursing/profanity, insensitive language, wastefulness, not being dependable or keeping promises, sarcastic remarks, gossiping, being disrespectful, irresponsibility, dourness, and negativity. And don't forget the Seven Deadly Sins: pride (vanity), envy, wrath, sloth, greed, gluttony, and lust.

People so often get away with these because of no perceived consequences, or at least not in the short run. In the end, though, their shenanigans often catch up with them. Absent legal consequences there still may be social consequences, especially when living in a tight-knit community where word of misdeeds travels fast. Reputation-protection is a strong incentive to avoid wrongdoing.

Legal and social repercussions and other worldly checks on behavior have their limits. Sometimes people could care less about their reputation or they aren't even aware they're doing anything wrong. Or there's a high likelihood no one else will ever know. It would be nice if everyone abided by Thomas Jefferson's dictum, "Whenever you do a thing, act as if all the world were watching." But they don't. With no one watching, only a sense of guilt may stop bad behavior. But that's by no means assured. What else could stop it? For an atheist or agnostic, not much. But for someone who believes supernatural agents are observing at all times, there's plenty of incentive to stay on the straight and narrow.

No less than God-basher extraordinaire Richard Dawkins even admits that. Known as one of the world's most famous atheists, Dawkins actually is an agnostic. He called himself one, admitting he can't be sure God doesn't exist.[2] He made a career out of thrashing religion, arguing it should be banished from society. Then he had a change of heart. Apparently appalled by the excesses of the growing secularization of society, he told *The Times* of London that the absence of religion would "give people a license to do really bad things." In the same way that an absence of security cameras invites shoplifting, "people may feel free to do bad things because they feel God is no longer watching them." He wrote in one of his books, "Whether irrational or not, it does, unfortunately, seem plausible that, if somebody sincerely believes God is watching his every move, he might be more likely to be good," he reluctantly admitted. "I must say that I hate that idea. I want to believe that humans are better than that. I'd like to believe I'm honest whether anyone is watching or not." He added that faith "might bring the crime rate down."[3]

Supernatural Supervision

Dawkins' newfound sentiments are backed up by rigorous scholarly research. Perceived supernatural entities encourage better behavior. Jesse Bering and colleagues tested this in a study at the University of Arkansas. Students enrolled in an introductory psychology course took a test in which it was easy to cheat. A portion of the test-takers were casually told that the ghost of a (fictitious) dead graduate student recently was seen in the testing room. (Two of them only agreed to participate if the door was left partially open while they were being tested alone in the room.) Compared with those who didn't hear the ghost story, participants who did hear it performed significantly worse on the test—i.e. they didn't cheat.[4]

While at the Institute of Cognition and Culture at Queen's University (Belfast) and a then-committed atheist*, Bering along with Jared Piazza and Gordon Ingram carried out another such experiment, described in their paper "'Princess Alice is Watching You': Children's Belief in an Invisible Person Inhibits Cheating." They divided sixty-seven youngsters ages five to nine into three groups, having them play a game where it was nearly impossible to win unless they cheated. They threw a ball at a Velcro dartboard, with strict rules. Only by skirting the rules such as manually placing the ball on the target could a child "win" and get a prize. One group was supervised, another was not, and another was told an invisible magic princess, "Princess Alice," was watching them. Several of the older children expressed disbelief in the princess—but not before manually feeling the chair where she was alleged to have been sitting, and waiving their hand through the air above it in an effort to ensure she wasn't really there.

The results? The unsupervised group cheated the most by far. The supervised group for the most part refrained from doing so. As for the Princess Alice group minus the skeptical children, you

---

* More recently he wrote in his *Scientific American* blog, "I'm not quite ready to say that I've changed my mind about the afterlife. But I can say that a fair assessment and a careful reading of (Ian) Stevenson's work has, rather miraculously, managed to pry it open. Well, a tad, anyway."

guessed it: they were just as likely to not cheat as those in the group supervised by a real human.[5]

All too often, people engage in unethical or criminal activity because they know they have a very low chance of getting caught. They think no one is looking. By contrast, the deeply religious think someone always is looking whether it be God, angels, devils, saints, or souls of the dead. In Judaism, Christianity, and Islam it's believed God not only is always watching you but knows your intentions and motivations. He's fully omniscient; not just your good deeds but also your every sin in thought, word, and deed are being recorded for judgment in the afterlife. In Hinduism and Buddhism, through karma, it's thought that violating moral codes has negative consequences either in this life or future lives. Even in shamanism, evil spirits are always said to be lurking about, ready to inflict punishment on anyone who displeases.

"God knows what you did. God is going to punish you for it. And that's an incredibly powerful deterrent," Dominic Johnson of the University of Edinburgh told a National Public Radio correspondent. "Everywhere you look around the world, you find examples of people altering their behavior because of concerns for supernatural consequences of their actions. They don't do things that they consider bad because they think they'll be punished for it."[6]

Mercy Yet Justice

Rising crime, vice, immorality, and churchlessness in society stem not only in part from ever-increasing atheism, but also from the widespread belief that God is only love and mercy. Whatever wrong you do, it's thought, you'll be forgiven and go straight to heaven. He certainly is loving and merciful, but full of justice as well. A rigorous and demanding God is not just found in the Old Testament. In the Gospel of Matthew in the Sermon on the Mount as well as elsewhere in the New Testament, Jesus displays plenty of rigor. For example,

"You have heard that it was said to your ancestors,

'You shall not kill; and whoever kills will be liable to judgment.' But I say to you, whoever is angry with his brother will be liable to judgment. (Matthew 5:21-22) …You have heard that it was said, 'You shall not commit adultery.' But I say to you, everyone who looks at a woman with lust has already committed adultery with her in his heart. (Matthew 5:27-28)…And if your right hand causes you to sin, cut it off and throw it away. It is better for you to lose one of your members than to have your whole body go into Gehenna." (Matthew 5:30)

Gehenna is a reference to hell and is often translated that way. Jesus mentions hell either directly or indirectly some sixty times in the Gospels. By contrast, in the Old Testament, Sheol or the place of the dead is mentioned more sporadically and is not even necessarily a place of punishment.

If everyone goes to heaven, why shirk from wrongdoing if you can get away with it? Why not indulge in vice? Why bother to go to church? Knowing that God is full of justice in addition to mercy is good for individuals and for society. Evidence backs that up. In their study "Mean Gods Make Good People," the University of Oregon's Azim Shariff and University of British Columbia's Ara Norenzayan showed that belief in a judgmental, punitive God prompts less cheating than belief in an exclusively loving, forgiving God. In two separate experiments, several dozen undergraduates from a variety of religious beliefs or non-belief took a math test in which it could be observed whether they cheated. Upon completion they were asked about their religious views and perception of God. The researchers found no difference in cheating between atheists/ agnostics and believers in an exclusively loving and forgiving God. There was significantly less cheating among students who considered God to be punishing and justice-minded. The researchers write, "Successfully enforcing honesty may not depend on the belief in just any supernatural agent but may require deities who are able to elicit credible fears of punishment. In other words, how much you believe in God matters less than what kind of God you believe in."[7]

Said Shariff, "Of course there's more to morality than not cheating. It's not clear from these data that punitive gods encourage more of this pro-social behavior (charity, generosity, etc.). What they just seem to do is reduce these kinds of negative aspects—antisocial behaviors. So it's a carrot and a stick. If you want to prevent people from doing (bad) things, it's usually more effective to use a stick, in this case the punitive God. It might be the case that if you're trying to encourage people to do positive things, a carrot might work better—a loving God."[8]

The perception a higher power is always monitoring you is particularly effective when it's associated with an organized religion that has a prescribed set of rules on moral behavior as well as rewards and/or punishments in response to that behavior. By contrast, without belief in a higher deity—or belief in a God of justice—there's less incentive to act virtuous. Certainly, atheists and agnostics have tools that promote ethical behavior. But Ted Turner's Eleven Voluntary Initiatives just don't hold the same sway as the Ten Commandments.[9]

No Pain No Gain

It often has been said that religion is a mechanism to control the people. In a sense that's correct, but not in the way the skeptics intend. It promotes control all right: self-control.

Self-control is the ability to quell short-term urges, desires, emotions, temptations, and behaviors to attain longer-term goals. It's the act of forgoing immediate comfort or pleasure in order to achieve a noble or worthy end. It's short-run pain for long-run gain. Or if not short-run pain, then at least short-run avoidance of something bringing no benefit later on.

Many studies confirm religious persons tend to have greater self-control/self-discipline than nonreligious. University of Miami scholars Michael McCullough and Brian Willoughby located thirteen studies on the relationship between self-control and religiosity. Twelve of them determined a definite positive correlation between the two.[10]

Self-control and specifically self-regulation is a "profoundly important topic of social psychological study," state Waterloo University's Kristin Laurin and colleagues, because it so affects mental as well as physical health, educational achievement, and overall well-being.[11] High-self-control individuals tend to have better: mental health, relationships, ability to accomplish tasks, and grades (as students).[12] Self-control even outweighs intelligence as a predictor of academic performance, as discussed in chapter 8.[13] Those with high self-control, moreover, experience lower alcohol and substance abuse and are less susceptible to crime and delinquency, suicide, risky sex, risky driving, viewing porn, unhealthy eating, and other negative factors. Religiousness is associated with self-control-related personality traits such as agreeableness, conscientiousness, and low psychoticism. And religious parents tend to have children with higher self-control.[14]

Unlike non-human mammals which generally lack the ability to control impulses, humans can ponder possible outcomes of certain actions and decide to undergo short-term pain or at least short-term denial for long-term gain. This is reflected in the large size of humans' prefrontal cortex—where self-control is mainly rooted—compared with animals of similar brain size. Good self-control, a.k.a. willpower, is key to success.[15] Religious practices activate the frontal lobes within which the prefrontal cortex is housed. This part of the brain is associated with empathy, impulse and emotion control, moral insight, optimism, hope, and having a sense of personal responsibility. As noted in chapter 2, brain-imaging studies indicate prayer and meditation stimulate the frontal lobes and increase blood flow to that area. This is consistent with prayer's correlation with better overall mental health, writes Patrick McNamara of the Boston University School of Medicine. Frontal lobe dysfunction, he reports, is associated with depression, impulsiveness, and drug and alcohol abuse.[16]

Greater self-monitoring results in greater self-control. This comes in part from perceived monitoring by supernatural entities, as well as by others who share your values and to whom you want to display those values. Also helpful are religious rituals and age-old practices. Confession for Catholic and Orthodox Christians, the season of Lent for Christians, and the Yom Kippur holiday for Jews involve examining thoughts and actions to discern sins and shortcomings. Factors such as these "may help explain why religious people tend to live slightly longer lives; suffer less from depressive symptoms; avoid trouble with sex, drugs, and the police; do better in school; enjoy more stable and more satisfying marriages; and more regularly visit their dentists," sum-up McCullough and Willoughby.[17]

Religiosity and specifically Christianity enhance self-control through teachings that certain thoughts and not just actions are sinful. For example, Jesus taught that "anyone who looks at a woman lustfully has already committed adultery with her in his heart." (Matthew 5:28) And "it is from within, out of a person's heart, that evil thoughts come—sexual immorality, theft, murder, adultery, greed, malice, deceit, lewdness, envy, slander, arrogance, and folly." (Mark 7:21-23) Five of the Seven Deadly Sins are "thought sins:" pride, envy, wrath, greed, and lust which easily can lead to "action sins."

Kristin Laurin of Waterloo University along with Duke's Aaron Kay and Gráinne Fitzsimons conducted an experiment measuring temptation resistance. Participants read a speech excerpt that either was about God (containing statements such as "God is the beginning and end of all things") or about the declassification of Pluto as a planet. They had to complete an evaluation form in the presence of a plate of bite-sized chocolate chip cookies which they were free to consume. As expected, the God-primed participants ate fewer cookies. And compared with those primed with neutral concepts, they had more negative automatic associations with foods such as potato chips, donuts, and chocolate. "These findings represent, to our knowledge, the first experimental evidence that thinking of God can improve temptation resistance even in domains unrelated to morality or religion, providing support for earlier theorizing about the beneficial impact of religion on self-regulation," declared the researchers.[18]

Meanwhile, people differ in their ideas of how omniscient God is. The devout typically view God as watching their every move and knowing their every thought:

> "He plumbs the depths and penetrates the heart; their innermost being he understands." (Sirach 42:18)

Others view Him as only concerned about their most significant actions and behaviors. In Laurin and colleagues' tests, those whose concept of God included high omniscience were more resistant to temptation. Other participants said they would be more willing to resist temptations only if they believed God to be omniscient and mindful of transgressions.[19]

Of course, heightened self-control doesn't just apply to the Judeo-Christian tradition. Bengi Oner-Ozkan of Middle East Technical University surveyed Turkish Muslim college students to discern the extent to which they consider the future in their decision-making. Sure enough, the more religious students scored higher. The study notes that this mentality is associated with academic success, problem-solving, planning ability, and delayed gratification.[20] In a study of Indonesian eighth and ninth graders, teachers reported that the more religiously observant had greater self-control.[21] The same was true for postgraduate Pakistani Muslims. When faced with temptation they often sought guidance by consulting scriptures.[22]

In their study "Religion Replenishes Self-Control," Kevin Rounding and colleagues of Queen's University (Canada) primed some test subjects with religious words (e.g. God, spirit, divine), others with neutral words, and others with morality-themed words (e.g. righteous, virtue) before having them carry out tasks measuring self-control. In psychology, to "prime" is to expose patients or research subjects to certain messages or information with the hope of it lingering in their minds so that when presented with another stimulus, the primed information affects their reaction. In the Rounding study, compared with the neutral words, exposure to religious words promoted self-control. Perhaps surprisingly, exposure to the moral words did not. "We consistently found that when religious themes were made implicitly salient, people exercised greater self-control, which, in turn, augmented their ability to make decisions in a number of behavioral domains that are theoretically relevant to both major religions and humans' evolutionary success," they write.[23]

Not all studies find a correlation between self-control and religiosity. In the wake of the Rounding study, two Australian scholars questioned his methodology—specifically how he measured self-control. So they sought to replicate his word-priming experiment with the self-control component adjusted. They found no association between test subjects primed with religious words, and self-control. They write, "We suggest that it is not the ability—but motivation—to delay gratification that is influenced by religious concepts."[24]

Another study found no correlation between self-control and those who place high importance on religion but who don't necessarily attend regular religious services. Even then, churchgoing isn't always associated with self-control. That's particularly true when the person is extrinsically religious.[25] This entails attending church mainly for social or cultural reasons rather than based on a strong belief in, and personal relationship with, God. (More on extrinsic religiosity in chapter 12.)

Scott Desmond of Indiana University-Purdue University Columbus in a 2008 study concluded that religiousness—as measured by frequency of prayer and church attendance as well as by personal importance of religion—is "positively and significantly" associated with various measures of self-control. But a more recent study of his ascertained that among adolescents, religious service attendance and the importance of religion were not significantly related to self-control. The religious teens, however, did indicate that it's less acceptable to break moral rules. They also are less likely to keep secrets from parents. In the same survey, teens identifying as "spiritual but not religious" had lower self-control and indicated it's more acceptable to break moral rules.[26]

A question arises whether religion engenders self-control, or whether people disposed to self-control tend to be more religious.

Lower self-control such as having attention deficit hyperactivity disorder might make it harder to sit through religious services and carry out the requisite beliefs and practices. So McCullough and Willoughby set out to evaluate already-completed studies related to that question. They found several that, taken together, suggest self-control leads to religiousness. But offering hope to those with ADHD and/or weak self-discipline, a study suggested religion precedes self-control. Experiments showed that when faced with temptation, the pious-minded may resist it by automatically invoking spiritual concepts in addition to prayer, scripture reading, meditation, and viewing/venerating religious imagery. And religiosity helps a person avoid temptation in the first place.[27]

When it comes to self-control/self-regulation, the psychological literature highlights two key elements: active goal pursuit, and temptation resistance. Active goal pursuit is just that—setting a goal and doing actions to reach that goal. If you aim to lose weight, active goal pursuit may entail taking the stairs every day instead of the elevator, whereas temptation resistance may be turning down that three-cheese bacon pizza and settling for a veggie sandwich instead. Someone could put more emphasis on temptation resistance than on active goal pursuit. That particularly may be the case when religion is involved. Laurin and colleagues found that while exposure to God concepts can bolster temptation resistance, it may weaken active goal pursuit. Some religious persons view events ultimately determined by the will of God, especially events out of their control or unexplainable, prompting them to think the impact of their actions is limited. Among certain people, the result could be less motivation for pursuing particular goals.[28] But that certainly doesn't apply to religious athletes, among others. As detailed later in this book in chapter 8, their faith instills in them more motivation to pursue their goals.

Sin and Society Revisited

In 1907 the book *Sin and Society: An Analysis of Latter-Day Iniquity* was published. In it, author Edward Alsworth Ross argued that the rise of big business, big government, and big media enabled new types and varieties of sins that didn't exist in pre-industrial times. "The cloven hoof hides in patent leather," writes Ross. The person who may seem like a well-dressed, upstanding member of society may actually, through greed or neglect, be taking actions or lack of actions at his place of work that result directly or indirectly in scores of people getting hurt or swindled. They included child labor, adulterated foods and goods, embezzlement, pollution, lack of factory safety measures, ballot-box stuffing, landlords who neglect safety, corrupt editors, "school-board grafters who blackmail applicants for a teacher's position," tax-dodgers, venal government safety inspectors, the government clerk who secretly reveals advance crop information, and the labor leader "who wields strikes as a blackmailer's club."[29]

Most of these fall under the rubric of white-collar crimes or unethical behavior. They're usually easier to get away with because they're less obvious than traditional crimes. How can those sins be stopped? With God watching their every move, people of faith know they'll be held accountable for their sins after they leave this world. That's a huge incentive to live as ethically as possible. With the rise of new occasions of sin owing to the transformation of society during Edward Alsworth Ross's time, it's certain that far less lawless and unethical behavior went on than otherwise would have, owing to the strong religious convictions of most people of that era.

Many of those sins have greatly diminished since Ross wrote his book, thanks in part to prudent government regulations, media watchdogs, greater transparency, and keen competition to produce the finest goods and services. But temptations and opportunities to commit them still abound. Not only that, but in the more-than century since the book was published, wholly new temptations and occasions for sin have flourished. Edward Alsworth Ross died in 1951. If only he had been around to see the proliferation of types and varieties of sins in the era following his death, due in part to advancements in technology, greater mobility of people and products, relaxation of certain laws, and weakening social norms.

We in today's society are blessed and cursed: blessed thanks to modern products and services that make our lives more comfortable and enjoyable; cursed because so many of them can be misused or overused. The Internet and other technologies as well as changing social norms and laws have given rise to innumerable sins that were rare or not possible in previous eras. They include pornography, social media abuse and misuse, cyberbullying, sexting, defamation via electronic dissemination, video game overuse, junk-food fueled gluttony, illegal drug use, prescription drug abuse, extramarital sex (facilitated by the birth control pill and other forms of contraception), abortion, and assisted suicide (the latter two facilitated by new medical technologies and procedures, as well as legalization). Never before in history have there been so many opportunities to sin. Never before has it been harder to avoid.

Take pornography for example. It was almost nonexistent until the invention of the camera. Then the twentieth century ushered in X-rated movie theaters in addition to magazines, followed by pornographic videotapes, pay-per-view television (which often showed up without having to pay), the Internet, and smartphones. Technologies enabling porn are so readily available to practically anyone that an estimated 65 percent of American men and 41 percent of women view porn at least once a month.[30] Several pornography websites are consistently ranked among the top-ten most visited websites in the world. And as someone once said, a child having a smartphone is like having an X-rated movie theater in his pocket.

In today's temptation-ravaged world, adults and kids alike must be ever-disciplined and resolute—much more so than in previous eras. We need self-control to resist peer pressure, to resist uttering that sarcastic or hostile remark, to resist that second bag of chips, to resist that extra drink. Same for raunchy movies and shows, clickbait, gossiping on social media, immodest fashion trends, and tapping into our hand-held movie theaters. It takes character and determination to not only avoid indulging in what's bad but also to discern what's good and what's bad. Robust self-control means better outcomes behaviorally, academically, emotionally, physically, financially, and spiritually.

Non-churchgoers are far less exposed to advice and information on resisting temptation. Secular society just doesn't offer that guidance very often. While secular sources dole out plenty of advice on resisting drugs, alcohol, and overeating, the range of subjects falls woefully short. Media shy away from certain things because they don't even consider them harmful, such as porn and other sexual sins. At the time of this writing a mainstream magazine—*Forbes*—even has a section called "Vices"; not condemning vice, but writing positively about it, mainly focusing on marijuana but also booze, gambling, and sex.

A simple Internet search of "resist temptation" shows that the vast majority of help in this area comes from faith-based sources. Religious traditions and practices are an additional motivator. During the Lenten season in Christianity for example, the faithful are encouraged to give up for forty days something they normally enjoy, such as sweets, snacks, video games, or televised sports. Mastering the self-discipline to deny oneself small things strengthens the ability to eradicate harmful habits. Being around others who keep tabs on you can have a significant effect as well, be they clergy, fellow congregants, youth ministers, or religious education teachers.

Among the biggest temptations in everyday life is to grumble, gripe, whine, and lash out. Especially when tired and hungry, we could be impatient and edgy, ready to pounce on real or perceived slip-ups from spouse, kids, siblings, friends, workmates, or anyone else around us. To combat this, the pious may think of the Golden Rule or say a prayer or two. When drawn to contempt or hatred, they may recall teachings on the importance of forgiveness, and love for enemies. When drawn to lust, they may hark back to teachings that the body is a temple of the Holy Spirit and avoid doing anything to profane it. When drawn to covetousness, they may summon up teachings that only God can ultimately satisfy the heart.

A team of eight researchers led by Everett Worthington of Virginia Commonwealth University found that compared with those of low religiosity, people of high religiosity tend to employ more robust strategies to resist or suppress sexual attraction to those other than spouse or significant other. Strategies include physically or mentally avoiding the attractive person, or thinking of the attraction as inappropriate including invoking religious teachings.[31]

The faith-filled also are better at resisting porn. Mary Short and colleagues at the University of Houston-Clear Lake confirm that religiosity is associated with less pornography consumption—particularly intrinsic (i.e. highly devout) religiosity. They also report that shunning pornography corresponds with lower levels of depression and more satisfactory marriages, and for single persons, a better understanding of who they want in a dating relationship.[32]

Slippery slopes to sinful action abound. Strong religious belief helps in steering clear of boundaries beyond which temptations lurk, such as alcohol-fueled parties, racy movies, racy websites, casinos, and pals liable to lead you astray. When bumping up against a boundary several times, human behavior is such that one of those times the self-control breaks down. "A boundary that may be safe for us one day may be hazardous to us the next, depending on our emotional state," writes Joseph Tkach at Grace Communion International's website. "So a boundary, if it's going to work, has to be set for our weakest moment, not our strongest."[33] A person may be able to resist indulging in a certain sinful pleasure 99 times out of 100. But during a moment of weakness the boundary is breached. That's why, adjacent to the boundary it's important to set up a buffer zone in which not to tread.

Not all temptations are created equal. What leads one person into temptation could be perfectly fine for another. For example Mike attends his buddies' poker game, loses $20 and has no problem stopping and cutting his losses thanks to his strong sense of self-control. Bob on other hand keeps trying in vain to win back his money and digs himself deeper into a hole, losing a few hundred dollars that could have been put toward his kids' education fund. Bob's buffer zone is the poker game or casino—best not even to get within ten miles of either. When offered a beer at the bar with

coworkers, Mike is fine with one or two. Bob downs them one after another. Mike clicks links to news stories in websites with racy
pictures plastered up and down the right-hand margin, just reading
the news while not even glancing anywhere else. Bob by contrast
succumbs to the clickbait quickly.

It's easier to resist sin when we know someone is keeping tabs on
us, whether they're bodily or spiritual beings. In the bodily domain,
churches and other faith-based organizations often sponsor men's
or women's groups in which each person has an accountability
partner. This is someone to meet and/or communicate with regularly to confidentially discuss challenges and report on progress in
overcoming temptations. An accountability partner also could be a
pastor, co-worker, friend, elder, spiritual director, or professional
counselor. For Catholic and Orthodox Christians, the sacrament of
confession is essentially an accountability session.

Through accountability partners, Bible teachings, and sermons,
along with faith-based motivational speakers, books, and websites,
the faithful are in a better position to learn about and combat temptations than the nonreligious. It's yet another reason why churchgoers experience less depression, alcoholism, drug addiction, porn
addiction, divorce, suicide, and physical health problems.

Chapter 6

COUPLES WHO PRAY TOGETHER STAY TOGETHER

On his thirty-ninth wedding anniversary, speaker and author David Housholder reflected on what makes his and his wife Wendy's marriage strong. He discussed the importance of being cheerful, finding out the other's needs, living below one's means, and Sunday worship. "My wife and I have always been committed to going to church, even when we are on vacation. There is something about being physically present as a couple with a group of people who have set their intentions on living good lives and cultivating good relationships and being loving and kind with each other…It's like going to the gym, spiritually speaking." A couples group at their church meets every other week, and those couples have done "an awful lot" to enhance David and Wendy's marriage. The pair see marriage as a sacrament, as something bigger than the two of them; "…seeing marriage as an institution which is sacred, something which is indissoluble. It's something you can't take apart. It's a permanent marker."[1]

David and Wendy's faith fosters their marriage, and marriage fosters health. Churchgoers do better physically and psychologically because they're more likely to tie the wedding knot, their relationships are sounder, and they divorce less.[2] They have higher marital satisfaction. They resolve conflicts quicker. They communicate and collaborate better. They're less verbally hostile during disagreements. They're less prone to stalemates. And in line with David Housholder's reflections, they often view their marriage as sanctified.

Abundant studies confirm that married people by and large are happier, healthier, have fewer serious illnesses, and live longer:

- "The size of the health gain from marriage is remarkable. It may be as large as the benefit from giving up smoking," trumpet Chris Wilson of the University of East Anglia and Andrew Oswald of the University of Warwick and of Harvard. They surveyed numerous studies on the health and wellness impact of marriage. Among the married, divorced, separated, widowed, and never-married, marrieds easily have the lowest risk of dying prematurely.[3]

- *The Longevity Project* (see chapter 1) reveals that married men live about a decade longer on average than non-married men; married women live about four years longer than their unmarried counterparts. Fewer than a third of divorced men made it to age seventy in that study. A larger portion of never-married men reached that age, and still more married men did.[4]

- Marrieds have a 14 percent lower risk of mortality than divorcees and a 10 percent lower risk than never-marrieds, according to two studies, one of which was a meta-analysis of fifty-three studies.[5]

- Married people are more likely to be satisfied than singles and divorcees, and the well-being benefits last into old age. During middle age, when many experience a dip in well-being, marriage makes the dip less pronounced.[6]

- A report prepared for the Department of Health and Human Services by Mathematica Policy Research, Inc. surveyed various studies on marriage, and while the researchers found both positive and negative effects, they did say marriage is linked to improvements in mental health for both men and women. It also tends to reduce heavy alcohol consumption and marijuana use among young adults. "There is also substantial evidence that growing up with married parents leads to better long-term physical health, particularly for men." As far as negatives, their data showed marriage may encourage a more sedentary lifestyle, with modest weight gain and reduced physical activity.[7] So get off your duffs, dads.

- Divorce takes a toll not just on mental but also physical health. Remarrying does tend to improve health and longevity compared with single persons, but not as much as compared with the once-married-always-married.[8]

• Needless to say, divorce takes a toll on children. Their educational and psychological outcomes, on average, are not as high as children of intact families.[9]

So it really pays to get and stay married and put God at the forefront. If you're married and not going to church much or at all, start going once a week as a couple. If your spouse won't go, then go yourself and bring your kids.

As one wife married twenty-five years testified, "We start the day with prayers...We don't get out of bed without praying and trusting God to take care of everything. We put God first in everything that we do."[10] Couples in long-lasting marriages often affirm that their faith strengthens commitment to each other in addition to helping them get through hard times. Spiritual activities help focus couples' minds on nurturing and sustaining their relationship, encouraging commitment and forgiveness. Religion provides meaning and purpose not only to life but to marriage.[11] It champions age-old virtues such as forgiveness, honesty, integrity, selflessness, and generosity. As author and humorist Robert Quillen is reported to have said, "A happy marriage is the union of two good forgivers."

VanderWeele told the *Christian Post*, "The religious community provides social support, a constant reinforcement and reminder of religious teachings, family programs, communal worship, and experience of God. I would not say good marriages need a (religious) community to thrive, but it certainly does help."[12] That's reflected in the following points:

• Churchgoing couples are 30 to 50 percent less likely to divorce.[13]

• After regular churchgoing early in marriage, ceasing to do so could lead to trouble down the road—a 2.5 times higher likelihood of divorce than if they had kept up the faith.[14]

• Those viewing their faith as "very important" are 22 percent less likely to divorce than when viewing it as "somewhat important."[15]

- The very religious are significantly more likely to have higher-quality relationships and be very happily married than somewhat religious or nonreligious couples.[16]

Surely, somewhat religious (who go to church once a month or less) must have better relationship quality than nonreligious, right? Wrong. The quality is lower on average than even the nonreligious. It's yet another reason to never skip the Sabbath.[17]

In the 1980s, Howard Bahr and Bruce Chadwick of Brigham Young University analyzed a survey of residents of Muncie, Indiana—dubbed "Middletown" by a larger ongoing study—and found that "the more religious residents of Middletown were more likely to be married, to remain married, to be highly satisfied with their marriages, and to have more children." Sixty percent of frequent attenders considered their marriages to be "very satisfactory" compared with 43 percent of seldom-attenders. Non-churchgoers were more apt to say they were "dissatisfied" or "very dissatisfied" with their marriage.[18]

When one spouse attends little or never, the higher the risk of divorce. BYU's Vaughn Call and Tim Heaton who analyzed data from the National Survey of Families and Households also found that the wife's religious beliefs regarding marriage and sexual fidelity have a larger influence on marriage stability than the husband's beliefs.[19] But a more recent study by sociology professors W. Bradford Wilcox of the National Marriage Project at the University of Virginia and Nicholas Wolfinger of the University of Utah unearthed that when only the husband attends worship services regularly, 78 percent of couples report being "happy" or "extremely happy" in their relationship, versus only 59 percent when the wife attends but not her husband. When both attend regularly it's 78 percent, versus 67 percent happy or extremely happy when neither attends.

As to what accounts for the difference in relationship quality between a wife-only-churchgoer couple and husband-only-churchgoer couple, Wilcox and Wolfinger speculate that churchgoing women may be disappointed in not experiencing spiritual communion with their husbands, whereas men may not be as emotion-ally affected. The churchgoing also may prompt women to have higher expectations for husbands, which the husbands don't live up to. Another reason could be that the difficult relationship came first, prompting the wife to start attending church in an effort to seek religious help. And the emphasis that religious institutions put on marriage and family could benefit husbands to a greater extent since it's they who typically devote less time and attention to family than do wives. Unfaithful spouses are more likely to be men than women, so religious services may positively influence men in that regard.[20]

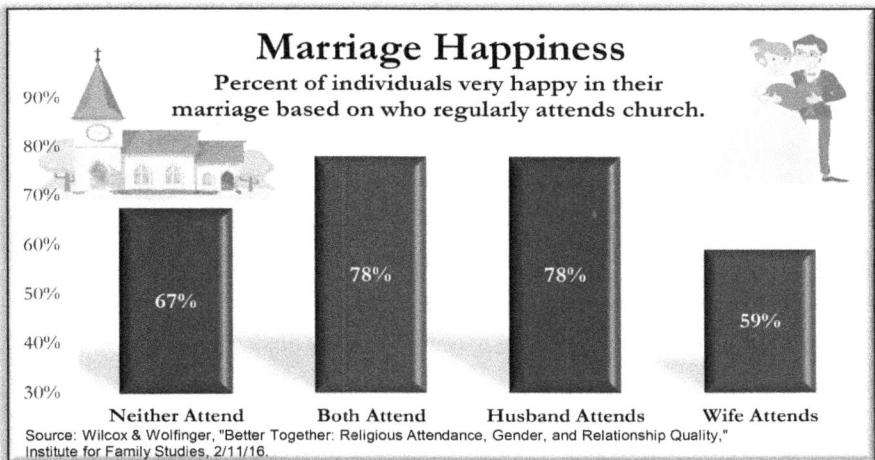

Marriage Happiness
Percent of individuals very happy in their marriage based on who regularly attends church.

Neither Attend	Both Attend	Husband Attends	Wife Attends
67%	78%	78%	59%

Source: Wilcox & Wolfinger, "Better Together: Religious Attendance, Gender, and Relationship Quality," Institute for Family Studies, 2/11/16.

So husbands, listen up: the more you plop yourself down in the pews, the more you'll ingratiate yourself with your wife. She'll be happier with the amount of time you spend together, and maybe even with your level of affection and understanding.[21]

Singles, boost your prospects of getting and staying married. Put on your Sunday best and head down to the building with the cross on top. Who knows—you may meet your future spouse there. And keep in mind that it helps to marry someone of the same religion or denomination. Several studies have shown that such couples argue less, have greater well-being, and report more marital satisfaction.[22]

The Religious-Nonreligious Divorce Rate Myth

There's an oft-heard claim that Christians divorce just as much or even more than atheists and agnostics. That may be the case if only taking into account people who call themselves Christians but don't attend church. Factor them out of the equation and just include regular churchgoers, and the Christian divorce rate is substantially lower than that of the unaffiliated.

American Christians' divorce rate is about 42 percent, compared with the religiously unaffiliated's 50 percent rate. University of Connecticut sociologist Bradley Wright deduced this by analyzing the General Social Survey compiled by the National Opinion Research Center at the University of Chicago. He also uncovered that at 38 percent, evangelical Protestants who attend church once a week have a lower divorce rate than Christians overall. But beware all you who call yourself evangelical yet repeatedly play hooky when it comes to church: your average divorce rate is 60 percent—considerably higher even than that of the religiously unaffiliated.[23] It's yet another stark reminder of the importance of regular public worship. A separate study found similar results: "nominal conservative" Protestants are 20 percent more likely to divorce than the religiously unaffiliated, according to Wilcox.[24] This refers to those who call themselves Christian—perhaps because their parents were

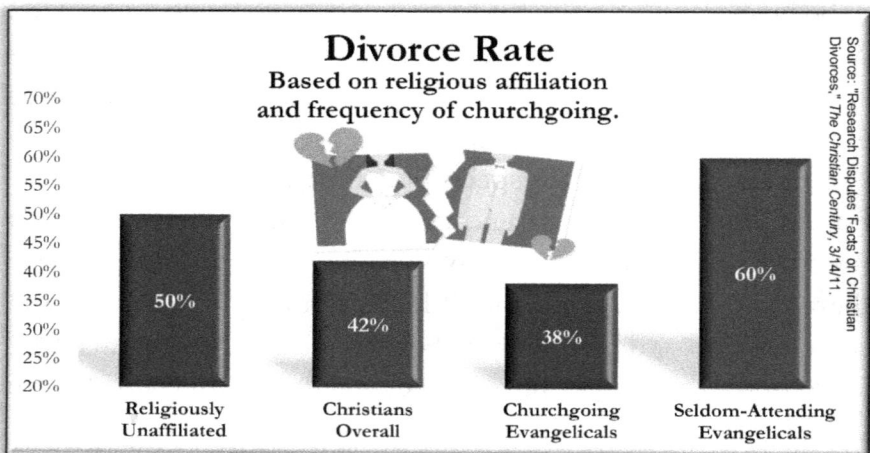

Divorce Rate
Based on religious affiliation and frequency of churchgoing.

70% 65% 60% 55% 50% 45% 40% 35% 30% 25% 20%

Religiously Unaffiliated	Christians Overall	Churchgoing Evangelicals	Seldom-Attending Evangelicals
50%	42%	38%	60%

Christian—but who rarely or never go to church. They typically are of weak faith, forfeiting the benefits of religion in maintaining a stable marriage. So in predicting the likelihood of staying married, it's religious attendance that's important, not religious affiliation.

Likewise, it has been said Catholic Christians divorce at a rate similar to the average U.S. divorce rate. The Center for Applied Research in the Apostolate (CARA) at Georgetown University puts this myth to rest. Its survey, covering 1972 through 2012, finds the percentage of U.S. adults who had ever married and experienced divorce was 36 percent. For Catholics it was 28 percent. For Protestants it was 39 percent, and for those with no religious affiliation, 42 percent.[25]

Also of note, Catholics who marry non-Catholics have a considerably higher divorce rate than Catholics who marry Catholics. Following is a breakdown:

Catholics who marry…	Divorce rate:
…Protestants	49%
…nonreligious	48%
…non-Protestant religious	35%
…Catholics	27%

The CARA survey doesn't indicate the divorce rate of regular churchgoing Catholics versus non-regular churchgoing Catholics. Based on the studies discussed earlier in this chapter, it's safe to say the regular attenders' divorce rate is significantly lower than that of infrequent attenders.

Whether Catholic or Protestant, Christians prone to skip Sunday worship, in addition to being more likely to get divorced, are more likely to stray. Even if you pray at home often and place high importance on your faith but don't go to weekly worship, you're at a higher risk for infidelity. David Atkins and Deborah Kessel of Fuller Theological Seminary confirmed this. Compared with regular churchgoers, praying people who seldom or never attend services are about *four times* more likely to have had an affair.

What is it about populating the pews that so discourages adultery? One reason, suggest Atkins and Kessel, is peer pressure. "An individual who is regularly attending services will have a network of relationships within the church, synagogue, or mosque...Having an affair risks that the infidelity could be revealed within the religious community, which could have consequences from shame and embarrassment to being ostracized or removed from the community." They add that while attending services the couple likely is hearing teachings on the importance of marital fidelity.[26]

The physically able who pray at home but steer clear of church, while they may consider themselves religious, actually aren't that religious. If they were, then they'd go to church—a basic, essential element of religiosity or at least Judeo-Christian and Muslim religiosity. While non-churchgoing Christians may find certain teachings of their faith attractive, they ignore other teachings—among them keeping holy the Sabbath as laid out in the Ten Commandments. They're known as "cafeteria Christians" who pick and choose which teachings to accept and which to ignore.

The Catholic Church certainly has its share of pickers and choosers. Even among those who regularly attend Mass, the majority are cafeteria-minded.[27] Far fewer in number are Catholics who earnestly try to abide by all of the precepts of the faith. Such persons take seriously the Church's teaching that marriage is indissoluble, and that divorce and remarriage is prohibited except in cases where the Church deems the prior marriage was never valid in the first place. They also adhere to the Church's prohibition of artificial birth control, opting instead for natural family planning. With NFP, couples wishing to avoid pregnancy abstain from sexual relations during the fertile phase of the wife's menstrual cycle, using fertility-monitoring technologies to determine when that is.

The divorce rate of couples who practice NFP is incredibly low. A study by Richard Fehring of Marquette University and Michael Manhart of Couple to Couple League International disclosed that the odds of divorce for women who've practiced NFP are 58 percent lower than women who've never done so. The authors write that "Use of periodic abstinence with NFP is the practice of marital chastity and is thought to strengthen the marital relationship."[28] Another study by Mercedes Arzú Wilson of Family of the Americas Foundation compared Catholics who use NFP to Catholics who don't. She determined the divorce rate among NFP users ranges from an astoundingly low 0.2 percent to 3 percent. That compares with 7 to 15 percent for the other Catholics.[29]

Why is divorce among NFP couples so rare? First of all, if they practice NFP they're likely to take the other teachings of the Church very seriously, e.g. that marriage is indissoluble. Second, it has been suggested that NFP-practicing couples enjoy better communication and have a greater likelihood of seeing each other as equal partners, since NFP prompts both husband and wife to be more in tune with the natural cycles of the wife's body.

By contrast, contraceptives can weaken the marital bond. Without fear of pregnancy, contraception makes it far easier to have multiple sex partners prior to marriage. Knowing a spouse had multiple partners can be a cause for tension. Contraception also facilitates adultery, in which the cheating spouse has little fear that pregnancy will result from the illicit affair. It also can generate mistrust, when one spouse suspects the other is cheating, whether or not he or she actually is.

Buttressing the Marriage Bond

Anyone with a healthy faith naturally would conclude that strong marriages are thanks to God's graces. If you praise and worship Him and abide by His teachings, He'll repay you in kind. When long-married couples reflect on the key to their success, divine inspiration is frequently cited. "To me, it would be like being inside a room with no air, not to have God in a marriage," said one spouse.[30]

Other faith-based bonds include the elaborate rituals associated with religious wedding ceremonies, reinforcing the strong emphasis churches place on marriage. And through preachers, teachers, and the Bible, the faithful are exposed to messages on the importance

of marriage as well as the ignominy of going astray. Relevant Bible
passages include:

> "That is why a man leaves his father and moth-
> er and is united to his wife, and they be-
> come one flesh." (Genesis 2:24)

> "He who finds a wife finds a good thing and ob-
> tains favor from the Lord." (Proverbs 18:22)

> "Marriage should be honored by all, and the mar-
> riage bed kept pure, for God will judge the adulter-
> er and all the sexually immoral." (Hebrews 13:4)

Ways that married persons abide by such teachings include
setting up boundaries—for example by physically or psychologically distancing themselves from those they otherwise would find
attractive. This also entails avoiding websites and other media that
may feature pictures of scantily clad people which in turn could
degenerate into pornography, and/or wandering eyes. Avoiding
what in Christianity is called "the near occasion of sin" is key, i.e.
steering clear of settings which could lead to sin.

At church, couples often are in contact with others who formally
or informally act as monitors, mentors, and advice-givers, and offer
support and encouragement to those with relationship or family
difficulties. A community of worshipers also has many couples who
act as role models for younger couples.[31] For singles, churches can
facilitate courtship and eventual marriage by providing a forum in
which like-minded singles meet. Married members of the church,
meanwhile, are role models for them—diminishing fears or concerns about married life.

A person may be reluctant to marry his or her partner because
of doubts over whether the partner is responsible enough to raise
a family. Other concerns include infidelity, alcohol abuse, drug
abuse, or domestic violence. Strong adherence to religion tempers
the propensity to engage in such abuses, instilling confidence the
other partner will avoid them. Once married, the religious are more

disposed to have higher regard for the institution of marriage and therefore be less willing to divorce.

Those committed to marriage on religious grounds have more resources to draw from in enhancing the relationship and working through problems. This includes theologically grounded virtues and guidelines for dealing with conflicts as they arise. One or both spouses may for example make a concerted effort to invoke what are known in Christianity as the twelve Fruits of the Holy Spirit: charity, joy, peace, patience, kindness, goodness, generosity, gentleness, faithfulness, modesty, self-control, and chastity. As Tony Merida, author of *Christ-Centered Conflict Resolution*, remarked, "In our peacemaking, we're seeking to follow the way of our Lord; we're seeking to bring peace where there's strife, reconciliation where there's alienation, gentleness where there's hostility, reason where there are outbursts of anger, and mercy where there's opposition."[32]

Of course, simple prayer is a key ingredient. Whether married or unmarried, those who pray for their significant other tend to be more solidly committed. Florida State's Frank Fincham and the University of Georgia's Steven Beach did a study of undergraduate students in romantic relationships, as well as married African American couples, finding that "partner-focused petitionary prayer" leads to stronger commitment and better relationship quality. They stress it has to be partner-focused; self-focused prayer wasn't associated with increased commitment.[33] And according to another study by Fincham and colleagues, partner-focused prayer leads to better cardiovascular health for married persons, including "significant improvements in coronary perfusion, decreased left ventricular work, and increased coronary blood flow."[34]

At-home prayer and/or scriptural study can enhance bonding between the married persons as well as instill a sense of divine support, guidance, and purpose, according to UT San Antonio's Christopher Ellison and colleagues. Whether married or unmarried, regular prayer reduces the inclination to cheat. It also reduces conflict. "Couples who prayed during times of conflict tended to lower their levels of hostility and contempt, and they achieved greater openness and willingness to compromise and strengthened the sense of joint responsibility for problem solving and reconciliation," write the scholars.[35]

"Being religious is tantamount to being a good husband, a good wife, or a good parent, child or kinsman," observed Carle Zimmerman of Harvard.[36] And when things get rough, religion helps hold couples together. Financial, medical, and other crises can stress a nonreligious couple's marriage to the breaking point. Similar crises besetting a religious couple, knowing they're spiritually bound to each other, may have a smaller adverse effect.

Relationship professionals widely agree that the most important factor in keeping a marriage intact is commitment—to each other and to the institution of marriage. Many people are under the impression romantic love is the most important ingredient. An oft-cited reason for divorcing is "falling out of love." Couples with a stronger relationship, by contrast, realize the initial feelings of love won't necessarily endure and that ups and downs are inevitable. Something they have that divorcing couples lack is commitment. What helps solidify it? The initial wedding ceremony is a big one. The planning for the event, the expense, the relatives and friends there to witness it, the rituals, and above all the vows drive home the point to the couple that they've entered into something requiring commitment. So does the state-sanctioning of the marriage and any tax and other state benefits associated with it. But cultural norms conveying that it's a long-term commitment still aren't enough. Bolstering that message is the religious aspect. Being cognizant that you're making marriage vows in front of God—and not just in front of people—serves to strengthen commitment.

Sanctifying the Spousal Relationship

Religious couples enjoy an additional bonding factor that nonreligious couples lack: a belief their marriage is sanctioned by a divine authority. Sanctification in couples is defined as "a process via which the spouse or marital union is perceived as having divine character or sacred significance. Specifically, it is believed that God is an active partner in the marriage, and spouses tend to ascribe sacred qualities to the relationship or to their partners," according to Ellison and colleagues in their "Sanctification, Stress, and Marital Quality" study.[37]

Sanctification in the theological sense connotes transforming a worldly phenomenon into something sacred or divine. Or it simply could mean giving spiritual significance to a goal or other aspect of life. "Part of the power of religion lies in its ability to infuse spiritual character and significance into a broad range of worldly concerns," write Annette Mahoney, Kenneth Pargament, and Nichole and Aaron Murray-Swank at Bowling Green State University.[38] When married in a church, especially if you strongly believe in a higher power and in the spiritual authority of your church, you may consider your marriage to be blessed by both spiritual and church authorities. It's plain to see that anything of yours you consider to be sanctified or have transcendent significance is something you'd be very reluctant to part with.[39]

Judeo-Christian weddings establish a three-fold union of the couple and of God. Marriage is looked upon as being imbued with transcendental love and grace, with God being an active third party. In Hinduism, marriage as well as childbearing are viewed as being an important stage of spiritual evolution, and a means to enhance divine righteousness and morality, i.e. dharma.

Spouses who view their marriage as sacred and as manifestations of God and/or who see in it a divine purpose have less conflict, better conflict resolution, and better marital adjustment. That's what Mahoney and colleagues ascertained after combing birth registries to locate couples who had had a baby within the previous six to twenty-four months. They queried ninety-seven of them regarding their relationship, level of religiosity, and extent to which they considered their marriage as sanctified. "Greater joint religious activities and perceptions of marriage having sacred qualities were associated with less reliance by both spouses on verbal aggression and stalemate strategies to handle marital conflict," they write. "Spouses who view their marriage as having sacred, transcendent qualities may be more willing to forgive and accept their partners, more likely to minimize or dismiss minor conflicts, and more likely to engage in attributional processes and behaviors to resolve marital conflict effectively, and more likely to make greater use of religious coping methods."[40]

With household financial matters such a common area of stress, Ellison et al. revealed that ascribing sacred significance to a marriage helps couples better cope with these problems, not only through managing negative emotions but also through solving the issue at hand. They're also more inclined to treat economic hardship as part of a larger divine plan, and as an opportunity for personal growth.[41]

Sanctification fosters altruism and empathy, which can result in more frequent compliments and acts of kindness, better collaboration and negotiation, forgiveness, and less criticism and negativity. "The perception of divine presence in the relationship may help spouses come to see the best in their partners, to accept basic personality differences that make them unique, and to focus on their good intentions and desirable attributes," write Ellison and colleagues. The stronger bonding that comes with sanctification manifests itself in spending more time together in leisure pursuits, conversation, and other activities—and last but certainly not least, in a more rewarding sex life.[42]

Holy Rollers Have the Best Sex Lives

Modern, sexually liberated individuals—as opposed to those Bible-believing prudes—must have the best sex lives, right? Wrong. The Sex in America study conducted by researchers from the University of Chicago and SUNY Stonybrook found that conservative religious women generally enjoy higher sexual satisfaction.[43] The World Family Map Project in its annual report indicated that compared with less-religious or nonreligious married couples, highly religious ones enjoy significantly higher relationship quality and sexual satisfaction. Women in such marriages are about 50 percent more likely to be strongly satisfied with their sexual relationship.[44]

Sexual satisfaction is particularly robust for couples who practice natural family planning. What? That's another paradox. How can they have such good sex lives when they need to abstain from it ten or more days out of the month? Because, in the same way folks savor a gourmet meal after starving themselves all day, sexual abstinence prompts couples to more greatly anticipate, appreciate, and cherish the times when they do have relations. Research has shown that compared with using contraceptives, NFP enhances intimacy, sexual desire, and satisfaction. Those using the birth control pill, according to studies, have lower sex drives than those using NFP.[45]

During abstinence the couple may express their love in nonphysical ways such as date nights and intimate dinners. "The times of abstinence with NFP are an opportunity for greater communication," wrote a Catholic husband. "There are many couples I know who are so focused on the physical that they do not spend enough time on the emotional, mental, and spiritual aspects of their relationships."[46]

With contraception, communication and emotional bonding may be weaker. As Pope Paul VI wrote in 1968, "Another effect that gives cause for alarm is that a man who grows accustomed to the use of contraceptive methods may forget the reverence due to a woman, and, disregarding her physical and emotional equilibrium, reduces her to being a mere instrument for the satisfaction of his own desires, no longer considering her as his partner whom he should surround with care and affection."[47]

Cohabitation and Divorce

There's a common misconception that living together prior to marriage results in stronger marriages, since by doing so the couple could discern if they're compatible in a household setting. Those deemed to be so would then get married, and presumably continue their harmonious relationship until death do they part. Not surprisingly, it doesn't always work out that way. Married couples who cohabited before marrying have a 1.37 times higher divorce rate than couples who didn't cohabit, according to Stanford researchers Michael Rosenfeld and Katharina Roesler. Another study disclosed the likelihood of divorce is 59 percent higher.[48]

Why is this so? For non-cohabiters, marriage is more looked upon as a kind of sacrosanct license to share a bedroom and raise a family together; a big stepping stone that changes those newlyweds' mode of living in a major way. By contrast, when a cohabiting couple gets married, their living arrangement is hardly changed. For them, marriage typically doesn't have the same level of transformational clout that it has for a non-cohabiting couple. When times get rough, the "glue" isn't as strong and sacrosanctity is weaker, so they split. Also prompting a higher divorce rate is "relationship inertia." Since the couple is settled in the same abode, cohabitation makes it harder to break up before marriage, prompting couples to stay together who may not be compatible, and forfeiting finding a more suitable partner.

Rosenfeld and Roesler determined that for couples who cohabited, the likelihood of divorce isn't higher during the first year of marriage, but is higher in subsequent years. The divorce rate for non-cohabiting couples in fact was slightly higher than for cohabitors during the first year, 4.1 percent versus 3.9 percent. This likely is because of the sudden change in lifestyle for the non-cohabiters, which some find hard to get used to. However, their marital dissolution rates steadily fell after that. By contrast, cohabiting couples reached peak marital dissolution between two and five years after marriage. And compared with married couples in which the wife had cohabited only with the future husband, the divorce rate was "dramatically higher" for couples in which the wife had cohabited with someone other than the future husband.[49]

The less religious are much more likely to cohabit than their more religious peers, according to Arland Thornton, William Axinn, and Daniel Hill of the universities of Michigan, Chicago, and Toledo respectively. Likewise, cohabiters consider religion to be of lower importance than non-cohabiters.[50] Their study was published in 1992; no recent similar studies can be found. Were the same study carried out today, the numbers may be different but probably not by much. The researchers unearthed that:

- Parents' religiosity affects sons' and daughters' decisions to cohabit. For those whose mothers attended church several times a week, the cohabitation rate is only half the rate of those whose mothers never attended.

- Young women who attend church less than once a month cohabit at a rate over three times higher than once-a-week attenders.

- Young women who seldom or never attend cohabit at a rate seven times higher than several-times-a-week attenders.

- Prior to cohabiting, fewer than 20 percent of cohabiters attended weekly services. Once they cohabit they tend to steer clear of church altogether. "Many of these people experienced dramatic reductions in their religious attendance, presumably as a result of the decision to cohabit without marriage," write Thornton, Axinn, and Hill. Conversely, not cohabiting before marriage increases the odds of embracing church.

So cohabitation tends to make people less religious. Perhaps it's because they know cohabiting is a sin and are reluctant to go to church. Or they may decide their church teachings are wrong. Or, one partner could be less religious or nonreligious, negatively influencing the other partner's willingness to attend church.

It comes as no surprise that cohabitation is associated with higher rates of depression—both for the couple and for the kids if they have them. Even worse for the kids is when their parents never tie the knot at all, which is so common nowadays. Compared with marrieds, the couples by and large have higher alcohol abuse. Their relationships are lower quality on average, and they perceive significantly less relationship stability.[51] The children are more likely to suffer emotionally and educationally. By age twelve, their cohabiting parents are twice as likely as married parents to have separated.

The cohabitation surge is deadly alarming. In a report on the importance of marriage, eighteen scholars sounded off, "The rise of cohabiting households with children is the largest unrecognized threat to the quality and stability of children's family lives."[52]

Chapter 7

FAITH FOSTERS STRONG FAMILIES

In 1977, university professors Nick Stinnett and John DeFrain placed notices in four-dozen newspapers in two-dozen states that read, "If you live in a strong family, please contact us. We know a lot about what makes families fail; we need to know more about what makes them succeed." Responses poured in. The Family Strength Research Project was born. Stinnett and DeFrain mailed questionnaires to more than 3,000 who responded to the notice, asking them what traits made their families that way. Six were mentioned time and again. "Spiritual wellness" was one of them—cited by some 84 percent of the families. The other factors were high levels of communication, commitment, appreciation, time spent together, and ability to cope with crises.

"Spiritual wellness" entails regular church as well as love, compassion, sharing, and adherence to a moral code. Strong families express their spiritual dimension in daily life, and practice what they preach, wrote Stinnett and DeFrain. A head of a participating family remarked, "Our family has certain values—honesty, responsibility and tolerance, to name a few. But we have to practice those in everyday life. I can't talk about honesty and cheat on my income-tax return. I can't yell responsibility and turn my back on a neighbor who needs help. I'd know I was a hypocrite, and so would the kids and everyone else."[1]

Among students at UC Davis, the religious ones considered their homes and families to be happier, warmer, more accepting, and more communicative than those of nonreligious students. That's from a survey carried out in 1973 but for our purposes the results are still relevant.[2]

Dolores Curran, author of *Traits of a Healthy Family*, queried more than 500 professionals who worked with families, boiling down fifteen of the most common traits. Of those, "a shared religious core" figured prominently. She notes that secular society and the behavioral sciences fall short when it comes to teaching right from wrong, instilling respect for and service to others, and fostering a strong sense of family.[3] Religion conveys those values more powerfully—especially in the context of a continuously monitoring higher power. The Bible commands that parents be honored and obeyed (Exodus 20:12) and instructs parents to teach their children to love God (Deuteronomy 6:4-9). Sermons and religious education classes spread those messages. Religious bookstores and radio stations are filled with resources and advice on parenting. Churches sponsor activities that encourage family bonding such as retreats, camps, Bible study, and family-centered picnics and outings.[4]

In parent-child relationships, baptisms, circumcision ceremonies, and Hindu naming ceremonies confer spiritual meaning to the new life. Throughout childhood, invoking God and prayer can be a helpful calming technique during times of discord. Bedtime prayers expressing remorse and asking for forgiveness help keep God at the forefront of children's minds. Misbehaving kids are more likely to amend their ways when held accountable to not just their parents but a higher power. In the Catholic and Orthodox Christian faiths this is reinforced through the sacrament of confession, in which the child is obliged to confess his or her transgressions to God through a priest, who in turn typically offers guidance and advice regarding the misbehavior. During confession the child pledges to make "a firm purpose of amendment" so as to work to avoid repeating the sins, resist temptations, and replace vice with virtue.

"Being friendly, cooperative, a good listener, and handling anger well are all traits that contribute to high quality familial relationships," write Penn State's Lisa Pearce and UM-Ann Arbor's William Axinn in the *American Sociological Review*. "Thus the personal importance of religion should influence the quality of family relationships independently of, and perhaps more pervasively than, attendance at religious services."[5]

Parent-Child Bonding

Hey moms—want to have a strong bond with your kids, whether they're still at home or on their own? Embrace faith. In rating their relationship with their children, mothers who deem religion to be "very important" score substantially higher compared with mothers who don't. Pearce and Axinn analyzed the Intergenerational Panel Study of Mothers and Children, a thirty-one-year longitudinal survey of 1,113 predominantly Christian mother-child pairs in the Detroit metropolitan area. "The more important religion is to a mother, the more likely her son or daughter is to report a higher quality mother-child relationship," they write. This holds true even if the mother didn't embrace faith until during the child's upbringing. Conversely when mothers' religiosity declined during those years, so did relationship quality. Grandmothers play a key role as well. The study uncovered that the more religious they are, the better the rapport between their daughters and grandchildren.

It's important to maintain the child's religious involvement as he or she gets older. Relationship strength typically extends well into adulthood when both teens and mothers are regular churchgoers, according to Pearce and Axinn. When both mother and her eighteen-year-old son or daughter attend religious services with about the same frequency, their relationship tends to be "significantly better" five years later—according to mothers. However, the kids didn't always think so.[6] Well, at least the moms were happy.

As you'd expect, it's a similar story for dads. It had been thought that employment and income are key predictors of the extent to which fathers bond with children. But a stronger predictor is religion—thanks among other things to its emphasis on family as well as the family-centered social networks it engenders. Brad Wilcox's study, published in his book *Soft Patriarchs, New Men: How Christianity Shapes Fathers and Husbands*, confirms these findings.[7] In it he discusses several manifestations of stronger relationships that religiosity spawns. Churchgoing dads are more likely to have greater or more frequent:

- involvement in kids' education.
- volunteering in kids' activities such as scouting and sports.
- one-on-one interaction.
- sit-down family dinners.
- monitoring of their children.
- praise and hugs for them.
- time spent with them.

Observes Wilcox, "Compared to dads who say they have no religious affiliation, fathers who attend church regularly (several times a month or more) devote at least two hours a week more in youth-related activities, such as helping in Boy Scouts, coaching soccer, and leading a church youth group. Fathers who are regular churchgoers also report that they are significantly more likely to engage in one-on-one activities with their school-age children, such as helping with homework, reading to them, or playing a game, compared to fathers who do not attend religious services regularly. They are also at least 65 percent more likely to report praising and hugging their children 'very often', compared to unaffiliated fathers."[8]

Those Bible-totin' traditional dads always make their wives change the diapers and do the laundry, right? Wrong. Contrary to what one might expect, religious dads are more likely than nonreligious ones to agree that husbands should share childcare tasks and housework with their wives. That's based on a finding by Penn State sociology professor Valarie King in her study "The Influence of Religion on Fathers' Relationships with Their Children." It's consistent with God-minded dads' closer ties with their kids. "Religious men enjoy higher quality marriages, and good marriages pull men into relationships with their children, suggesting that for men, marriage and childrearing might indeed be a 'package deal'," writes King. She points out that certainly, plenty of nonreligious fathers have good relationships with their kids, as the faith factor is one of many things enhancing the parent-child bond. But she nevertheless affirms that based on her study, certain aspects of fatherly involvement are more common among the more religious, including:

- better-quality relationships with kids.
- positive expectations for their future.
- putting greater thought and effort into relationships.
- a stronger feeling of obligation to contact and/or visit adult children regularly.

Of her various measures, the only area where religious fathers were about the same as nonreligious fathers was providing financial assistance to adult children.[9]

Faith and Family Dinners

As pointed out above, homes with religious fathers have more regular family sit-down dinners. These are more important for health and well-being than you might think. So often, family members do their own thing for meals. They eat alone at the table, unwilling to wait for others to show up. Or they chow down in front of a screen, while doing their homework, or on the go. They may get fast food on their own, or grab a bite at their friend's house. When done habitually, none of that is healthy either physically or emotionally.

Eating with the family means better nutrition thanks to fruits, vegetables, and fewer sugary drinks. It also means better communication with those at the table. That's important because especially in the age of social media when kids are with their phones all day with little opportunity to converse with parents, family dinners force everyone to be together without phones—assuming that rule is enforced—and have a normal conversation. This way, parents are much more in tune with what's going on in their kids' lives.

Benefits of regular family dinners are multifaceted. Numerous studies confirm that kids accustomed to this are less prone to:

- depression.
- mood swings.
- drugs and alcohol.

- eating disorders.
- being stressed out from homework.
- becoming obese.

They also get better grades, have higher self-esteem, and are better communicators. Girls particularly benefit from regular family meals, according to a study.[10]

Sanctifying Family

A doctor who adopted five daughters and raised them as a single parent saw his familial responsibilities in a divine light. He described it as an "answer to a completely new summons to growth... It is a call to grow into deeper union with God in total abandonment to His Will. It is to live as the incarnated instrument of the Lord in the role of single parenthood."[11]

As with marriage, giving spiritual significance to family relationships enhances satisfaction in numerous ways. It conveys there's more than just social, biological, and psychological dynamics but spiritual dynamics as well. "Believing that a family relationship is a holy gift may provide people with a special sense of good fortune and joy," affirms Annette Mahoney and colleagues at Bowling Green State. They point out that when God is viewed as playing a central role, people feel more secure in relationships with other family members and confident the relationships will endure. The sacred quality bolsters resilience in the face of internal strife, daily pressures, sickness, death, and other family crises. When one member views the family as sanctified, other members may follow suit. "Sanctification may enhance the intergenerational transmission of faith which, over the long term, may serve as a 'feedback loop' between parents and children that amplifies their respective individual spirituality," write Mahoney et al.[12]

Viewing family as sanctified motivates parents and kids to take a greater stake in those relationships and work harder to preserve them. It may involve investing more time and energy in family matters, perhaps sacrificing other things such as work, hobbies, entertainment, and/or sports. Family members may be more motivated to accept personality differences with other members, forgive their wrongdoings, and work to resolve or minimize conflicts and disagreements between spouses, parent and child, or siblings. "When family relationships flounder, those who sanctify these bonds may also be more willing to recognize the problems and be less defensive about change because of the high psychological and spiritual costs of losing these types of connections," observe Mahoney and colleagues. They add that threats to sanctified relationships could intensify efforts of religious coping such as prayer.

Mahoney et al. conducted surveys that sought to gauge levels of sanctification as well as the health of relationships. People indicated how strongly they agreed with statements such as:

• My marriage is a reflection of God's will.
• My role as a parent is a holy duty.
• In my role as a parent, I follow the teachings of my church.

Not surprisingly, the more respondents agreed with such statements the higher the marital satisfaction, the more investment in marriage and family, the less frequent any strife, and the greater the conflict resolution.

Mothers showing higher levels of sanctification in parenting report lower verbal aggression with their children such as yelling and name-calling. Sanctification also is linked to avoidance of harsh disciplinary practices such as corporal punishment, but only for parents who have a more liberal interpretation of the Bible. For those with a more conservative interpretation, level of sanctification was unrelated to frequency of corporal punishment. However, for those mothers, sanctification meant more frequent positive interactions with children. Mahoney et al. summed it up this way: "These findings illustrate how the sanctification of parenting reveals a more complex picture of the role that religion plays in parenting, especially use of corporal punishment, than global, single-item indices of religiousness such as one's religious affiliation or frequency of church attendance."

There can be downsides to sanctification. Notable are high expectations that get dashed. When marriage and parenting turn out to be harder than expected, feelings of spiritual failure may set in along with more anxiety and guilt than would otherwise be the case. That's particularly true if, owing to their attitude of sanctification, the individuals feel immune or invulnerable to problems that arise. Denying the problem could impede problem-solving. "Greater sanctification of marriage may heighten some couples' idealism about marital harmony, making it more difficult to admit and deal directly with serious conflict," write Mahoney and colleagues. An example is post-partum depression. "Those who place motherhood on a sacred pedestal may be even more reluctant to acknowledge and deal effectively with intense feelings of sadness and despair after giving birth."

What about sanctification without religion? For some people, particularly those drawn from the ranks of atheists and agnostics, humankind is their deity—or probably more commonly, nature is their deity (given that many nonbelievers tend to see humans as corrupting or polluting the rest of nature). For them, there's nothing supernatural or theological about what they consider sacred. "In such a case, family relationships may effectively replace supernatural powers (e.g., God, karma) as the ultimate sacred reality," say Mahoney et al. Does this secular sanctification of human relationships have similar beneficial psychological effects as theological sanctification? The researchers say that empirically, it's unknown whether the sanctification needs to be tied to a broader religious belief system for beneficial effects to occur.[13] But it's a good bet that it does.

Instilling the Faith in Your Kids

If you have children at home, you naturally want them to have good spiritual, physical, and mental health after they grow up and for the rest of their lives. One of the best ways to help ensure that is regular churchgoing with both you and your spouse in tow. Purdue sociology professor Brian McPhail carried out a study confirming that not surprisingly, adult children are least likely to be religious if both parents never attended worship services. They're somewhat more likely to embrace faith if one parent sometimes attended, even more likely if both parents sometimes prayed in the pews, and most likely if both parents regularly did so.

Dads, never neglect Sunday worship. Otherwise, according to a Swiss study, the odds your children will fall away from the faith are astronomically higher—even if their mother regularly attends.[14]

In instilling faith, it helps if both parents are the same faith. McPhail cites several studies concluding that individuals with parents who practice two different religions or denominations are somewhat less religious as adults compared with parents of the same religion or denomination. But differing religions is still better than a parent who's faith-filled and one who's not. So if you can't be the same faith as your spouse, at least both of you should go to Sunday worship, if only for the benefit of your kids' adulthood. This is crucial. Studies have shown that a big reason for non-religiosity of adult children whose parents were different faiths is that the parents attended church less frequently. Such parents also tend to place less emphasis on holiness in the home, with less-frequent prayer and scripture reading. And the children participate in religious education activities less often. The good news is that when parents of differing faiths habitually attend church, their children are almost as likely to be regular worshipers as adults, compared with when the churchgoing parents are the same religion, according to McPhail's findings. "Both are associated with above-average levels of religiosity," he writes.[15] And if you can't get your spouse to head for the steeple on Sundays, go anyway—it's still better than neither of you there.

Chapter 8

CHURCH IS GOOD FOR KIDS

Chris and Mark were each raised Catholic and had middle-class backgrounds. One lived in Illinois, the other in Pennsylvania. As teens, both played on their school's football team and described their friends as "jocks." Chris believed God is an "all-knowing, all-person being" who "influences everything you do in life." He felt close to God and prayed constantly. He looked to the Bible to shape his views of right and wrong. "There's not a day that goes by when I don't think of God or thank Him," said Chris. Mark, by contrast, believed in a higher power but thought everything in the Bible is "crap" and that Jesus was just a regular person good at attracting followers. Mark's family had stopped going to church because of all the complaints from him and his siblings. But he said his mom is still very religious and "believing in all that bull crap."

Which boy do you think got better grades? A quick look at their report cards tells all: Chris's is filled with As and Mark's with Cs.[1]

Kids from religious families not only are more likely to get better grades. They also tend to be better behaved and adjusted. They engage in socially deviant activities to a far lesser extent.[2] They have better social skills, better approaches to learning compared with children of less-religious families, better self-control, and lower impulsiveness. The last two traits overlap considerably. A child may refrain from doing something pleasurable in the short run, knowing such an action could harm others or himself in the long run. It could be holding her tongue after being slighted. It could be refusing to drink that beer or smoke that joint when pressured by peers. It could be exiting out of a video game after an hour rather than waiting for a parent to drag him away from the console kicking and screaming.

As early as 1929 it was found that length of Sunday school attendance was positively correlated with self-control.[3] Teens with a good sense of self-control, in turn, get better grades and have more desirable personality traits on a broad range of fronts. Overall they have better mental health, better interpersonal skills and relationships, drink alcohol and overconsume food to a lesser extent, and have higher self-esteem.[4] The National Longitudinal Study of Adolescent Health, commonly referred to as Add Health, is an ongoing survey of some 20,000 from throughout the United States who were in middle- or high school in the mid-1990s and who continue to be tracked. In addition to asking students how often they attend church and pray, the survey gleaned information on several indicators of self-control. IUPUC's Scott Desmond and colleagues analyzed the data and found religiosity and self-control in adolescents are indeed positively correlated.[5]

"Religion is good for kids," write Mississippi State sociologist John Bartkowski and colleagues. They analyzed the U.S. Department of Education-sponsored Early Childhood Longitudinal Study-Kindergarten Class which surveyed parents and teachers of more than 16,000 mainly first-graders on matters related to behavior, self-control, and respect towards classmates. "The religious attendance of parents and a cohesive religious environment in the home yield significant benefits for children's behavioral, emotional, and cognitive development...The children who are doing the best are in households where both parents attend worship services frequently." They also found that frequent parent-child discussions about faith often positively affect child development—but family arguments about that subject negatively affect development. Bartkowski et al. add that consistent with the adage that "it takes a village to raise a child," another vital component is involving the child in church-related activities so he or she interacts with and receives instruction from adults other than the parents, by which the parents' values are reinforced.[6]

Church itself is a place where kids learn self-control. They need it to sit through a service for an hour or more. It's normally inappropriate to talk, eat, be fidgety, walk around, or play video games. It's a place where mastering the art of poise is imperative.

On a broader level, religion cultivates in children the practice of delaying or avoiding things pleasurable in the short run with the expectation of being gratified later on with worldly or spiritual success. Delayed gratification could mean passing over candy in favor of fruit. Or turning down a video and doing homework instead. Or deciding against boozing it up with friends rather than risking getting caught, getting sick, or crashing the car. Kids good at delayed gratification and self-discipline tend to do better academically, socially, and economically years later.

"Religious young people…are more likely to complete their education because they haven't gotten pregnant, or dropped out, or haven't gotten delinquent and jailed, or haven't used drugs and become addicted," Harold Koenig said in a presentation to the Army Chaplain Corps. "They're more likely to complete their education. They're more likely to get a better job. They're more likely to be able to afford health insurance including mental health care. It just goes on and on."[7]

Mastery Over Marshmallows

There are few more prominent examples of delayed gratification than the famous marshmallow test. In it, a child sits at a table in front of a marshmallow and is given a choice either to gobble it up immediately or wait several minutes and eat two of them. The first study on this was in 1972. In 1990 the researchers followed up with the participants. Those who "passed" the test averaged 210 points higher on the Scholastic Aptitude Test (now officially known as the SAT) than those who ate it right away. They also were more likely to finish college, earn higher salaries, have lower drug and alcohol abuse, and stay out of prison. Even their body mass index was lower on average.[8]

As reported by Angela Duckworth and Martin Seligman of UPenn, one study found that four-year-olds better at delaying gratification generally enjoyed higher academic achievement and social adjustment a decade later. Another study sought to determine whether any personality traits are better predictors of academic success than grade point average or SAT scores. Among thirty-two traits (such as self-esteem, energy level, and extraversion), only one is a better predictor: self-discipline. Yet another study looked at students of equal intellectual ability, and why some were members of the Phi Beta Kappa honor society and others were not. The key factor was the degree of self-discipline (i.e. delayed gratification).

Duckworth's and Seligman's own study found that self-discipline predicts academic performance more robustly than IQ. They chose 164 eighth-graders as their research subjects. In addition to collecting reports from teachers, parents, and the students themselves on the latter's self-discipline profiles, the researchers gave them an IQ test along with a questionnaire on study habits and a task to gauge their ability to delay gratification. The results showed that self-discipline is highly correlated with:

• higher GPAs.
• higher scores on standardized tests.
• fewer school absences.
• earlier homework start time and more hours spent on it.
• less television watching.
• higher admission to selective high schools.

Students who improved their grades during the course of the year had self-discipline, not necessarily high IQ. The study's results affirmed that attitude eclipses aptitude. "Underachievement among American youth is often blamed on inadequate teachers, boring textbooks, and large class sizes," pointed out Duckworth and Seligman. "We suggest another reason for students falling short of their intellectual potential: their failure to exercise self-discipline." They cited society's emphasis on instant gratification. "We believe that many of America's children have trouble making choices that require them to sacrifice short-term pleasure for long-term gain, and that programs that build self-discipline may be the royal road to building academic achievement."[9]

Thomas Edison was right when he said genius is 1 percent inspiration and 99 percent perspiration. Whether it be at school or work, less-brainy people often outperform. This shows how important nonintellectual abilities are in getting ahead. They include motivation and self-discipline. To boost prospects of your child taking on these traits, take them to church each week.

Self-discipline and delayed gratification stand out not only in a secular sense where rewards are expected later in life but in a theological sense where rewards are anticipated for the next life. A child may consider short-term benefits of stealing or lying to be outweighed by long-term benefits not only on earth but also in heaven.

Fostering Education and Achievement

The start of this chapter discusses Chris and Mark. They were among thirty teenagers interviewed for a study on faith and academics carried out by Ilana Horwitz of Stanford. The interviews were a supplement to her analysis of a survey of 3,290 adolescents that was part of the National Study of Youth and Religion. She classifies youths according to their religiosity as Abiders, Adapters, Assenters, Avoiders, and Atheists, where Abiders are the most religious and Avoiders and Atheists the least.[10] Among those five groups, Horwitz found that at 3.21, Abiders have the highest average GPA and Avoiders the lowest with 2.92.

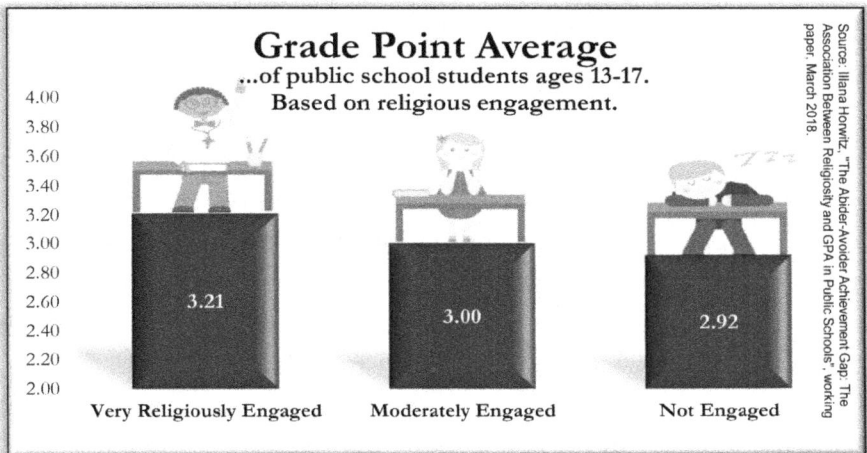

Grade Point Average
...of public school students ages 13-17.
Based on religious engagement.

4.00		
3.80		
3.60		
3.40		
3.20		
3.00		
2.80		
2.60	3.21	
2.40	3.00	2.92
2.20		
2.00		
Very Religiously Engaged	Moderately Engaged	Not Engaged

Source: Ilana Horwitz, "The Abider-Avoider Achievement Gap: The Association Between Religiosity and GPA in Public Schools", working paper, March 2018.

Note that next to Abiders, Atheists had the second-highest GPA. These are students who openly express disbelief in God, constituting just 3 percent of survey respondents. One can speculate they're more science- and/or activist-minded and thus study somewhat harder than the other three groups, nevertheless evidently are unaware of the abundant scientific evidence for God (see last chapter), a topic that unfortunately is avoided in classrooms for ideological reasons. Avoiders by contrast may consider there to be a God but show absolutely no interest in spirituality or religion—and evidently a less-than keen interest in their studies.

What accounts for the difference between Abiders and Avoiders? It relates to what scholars call religious social capital theory. Religiously engaged adolescents tend to develop habits highly valued in the public school system, namely conscientiousness and cooperation. Conscientiousness refers to being self-disciplined, organized, and achievement-oriented, while cooperation or agreeableness involves being considerate, kind, and sympathetic. In reviewing the interviews, Horwitz noticed Abiders spoke of experiences reflecting conscientiousness such as a boy refusing to take part in his friends' scheme at a fast-food restaurant to fill water cups with soda. Avoiders for the most part didn't recount such experiences and instead spoke of being rebellious, such as stealing clothes from the mall or making fun of teachers.

Some may argue conscientiousness begets religiosity rather than the other way around. Horwitz points out this is unlikely "because adolescents can't easily opt into or out of religious life—it is highly regulated by parents who socialize their children into their own religious systems."

It's no wonder that children of religious families on average have higher GPAs and standardized test scores. As summed up by the Marriage and Religion Research Institute, they tend to spend more time on homework, show up for class, take more advanced classes, have more academically oriented friends, and complete their curricula. Frequent churchgoing youth are five times less likely to skip school than their non-church-attending peers. They have fewer behavioral problems and are more likely to finish high school and get a college degree.[11]

While socioeconomic background and being on an academic/college track are the strongest factors in predicting academic success, religiosity is a significant factor as well. In addition to higher GPAs and standardized test scores, more religious students have higher expectations about future schooling. So found Mark Regnerus of the University of North Carolina at Chapel Hill who analyzed data from a national survey of tenth-graders as well as data from the Census Bureau. These relationships hold regardless of socioeconomic status, race, and gender. "Higher levels of involvement in church activities likely signifies, in addition to stronger family and community socialization, a level of social control and motivation toward education that leads to better math and reading skills," observed Regnerus.

One of his original hypotheses was religiosity mainly enhances academic achievement of adolescents from lower-income areas and not so much from middle- to high-income areas. He reasoned the latter typically have an abundance of extracurricular activities and social institutions that serve a similar purpose as religious institutions in promoting academic success. Low-income areas often have fewer opportunities for school clubs, sports leagues, scouting programs, and the like. When such programs do exist they're more likely to be affiliated with churches. Yet it turned out after he crunched the numbers, religiosity does significantly affect academic achievement among more well-off youth. Writes Regnerus, "This relationship between church activities and educational outcomes does not vary across income contexts, but rather appears to be important in all settings. Finally, while religious institutions may find themselves competing for students' time with school extracurricular activities, both of these integrating activities are related to schooling success."[12]

In a separate paper carried out with UNC-Chapel Hill's Glen Elder, Regnerus (then at UT Austin) notes that he's not suggesting the influence of religion is entirely social and easily replaced by secular activities such as little league baseball or scouting. Faith-based institutions are in a much better position to champion questions of right and wrong, drawing on the language of faith that secular institutions lack. "Religious communities prescribe and proscribe behaviors, organize initiatives, and sometimes even sanction individuals with the unique weight of moral imperatives."

Religiosity among high schoolers is associated with characteristics remarkably similar to those mentioned above regarding self-discipline, including:

• more time spent on homework.
• more advanced math courses.
• avoiding skipping classes.
• higher parental educational expectations.
• more discussion with parents about schooling.

The above comes from UT Austin's Chandra Muller and Christopher Ellison after analyzing a survey of high schoolers throughout the United States. They ascertained religious involvement is associated with more favorable outcomes among both the lowest- and highest-performing students. The results hold true for all racial groups.

Muller and Ellison tie religiosity to social capital, fostering such things as character and civic commitment. "Churches and synagogues are among the few institutions that sustain a coherent focus on issues of character, meaning, and purpose in life. This socialization may encourage young people to focus on 'big picture' concerns—what kinds of people they want to become, what long-term goals they have, and how best to accomplish them." Church-based activities expose youth to positive role models such as pastors, youth ministers, and religious education teachers, write the scholars. They also may cultivate friendships with peers who reinforce positive values including educational success.[13]

A large factor influencing outcomes is educational expectations of parents.[14] The more religiously involved parents are, the higher their expectations—and the more likely they are to talk to their kids about their education.[15] Within churchgoing families, children form a better conception of what their parents expect of them and thus are more prone to steer clear of areas such as alcohol and drugs, pre-marital and promiscuous sex, fights, truancy, and the like. Christian Smith of UNC-Chapel Hill points out that the more parents attend church, the more their children would perceive the parents to be upset with them if they dabbled in those practices. His study also found that religious parents supervise their children to a greater extent. The stronger the parents' religiosity the more they tend to know where their children are and how to contact them. They also have more rules. Smith concludes, "Accumulated scholarship provides ample empirical evidence that religion is a factor in the lives of American adolescents that often influences their attitudes and behaviors in ways that are commonly viewed as positive and constructive. In a number of areas of concern, different measures of religiosity are correlated with a variety of healthy, socially de-sirable outcomes."[16]

Even if they aren't religious themselves, many parents recognize that worship is good for kids not only spiritually but also moral-ly, socially, academically, mentally, and physically. So they fully embrace church and related activities, mainly for their children's benefit.[17] Those parents include atheist and agnostic scientists (both from the natural and social sciences) at elite U.S. universi-ties. Sociologists Elaine Howard Ecklund of Rice University and Kristen Schultz Lee of SUNY Buffalo deduced that about 17 percent of atheist faculty members with at-home children had attended a religious service more than once within the past year (versus 10 percent of nonparent atheists). They do so mainly to expose their children to a sense of community and to participate in religious rituals, as well as to instill a grounding in morality and ethics. Some of them don't want to inadvertently indoctrinate them with atheism so that the kids can make up their own minds what to believe when older.[18]

High school students attending church weekly or more have a .14 point higher GPA on average than those who never attend (for example 3.14 versus 3.0). Such concludes Jennifer Glanville of the University of Iowa along with David Sikkink and Edwin Hernández of Notre Dame who published their study in *The Sociological Quarterly*. One reason is churchgoing influences the friends one chooses, who tend to be more academically inclined. "Religious participation alters teen social networks, putting teens in greater contact with educational resources and pro-school values from peers. This may result from the simple fact that congregations can provide a social setting to meet and develop friendships with conventionally oriented teenagers," they write.[19] They also found:

• When parents know and interact with their children's friends and with the friends' parents—what academics call "intergenerational closure"—educational achievement is higher. Religious involvement encourages intergenerational closure which in turn promotes mentorship and role models. "Closure may facilitate better educational outcomes by facilitating norm enforcement and communication with other parents," write Glanville et al.

• Religiosity may boost involvement in extracurricular activities, especially non-sports activities, which in turn enhances academic achievement.

• Kids benefit by having to muster the discipline to sit still in church for an hour each week. This "may spill over into greater discipline in learning environments."

Churchgoing parents tend to structure their children's activities in ways that boost the likelihood of taking advanced courses and graduating from high school. Churchgoers end up having more years of schooling overall. In a 2004 study published in the *Journal for the Scientific Study of Religion*, Linda Loury of Tufts University analyzed the National Longitudinal Survey of Youth in which more than 12,000 were interviewed annually beginning in 1979. That year, 19 percent of them never attended church and 37 percent did at least once a week. By 1993 when they were in their early thirties, attenders averaged a half-year more schooling than non-attenders.

Faith-Based Schools

In addition to church, religious school tends to boost academic achievement. It also raises kids' social capital—the ability to build and tap into social networks to gain benefits and find solutions in life. They're less likely to be suspended, skip class, consume alcohol and drugs, be in trouble with the law, and engage in premarital sex.[20]

Prior to around the mid-1800s in America, education generally was run by religious institutions. Then, struggling religious-run schools increasingly turned to government tax money. Many transformed themselves into public schools, and new such schools were founded. By 1892 about 70 percent of U.S. high school students went to public schools. Religion was allowed to be promoted in public schools until Supreme Court decisions in 1962 and 1963 outlawed vocal prayer and Bible readings respectively. Schools even became hesitant to teach values such as love, forgiveness, turning the other cheek, and the Golden Rule for fear they were too related to religious teachings.[21]

Whether it was just coincidence with the no-prayer policy or not, in 1963 there began a nationwide decline in public school students' average standardized test scores as measured by the SAT and Iowa Assessments (formerly Iowa Test of Basic Skills) that lasted until the early 1980s before leveling off. It became apparent that Catholic and other faith-based schools were outperforming public schools. Education experts such as William Jeynes of CSU Long Beach questioned whether the absence of Judeo-Christian teachings in public schools could have negative behavioral and academic impacts.

To determine whether faith-based schools outperform public schools, Jeynes conducted a meta-analysis of ninety studies evaluating student achievement of religious, public, and charter schools. In addition to academic achievement and standardized tests, he took into account:

- The extent to which students are likely to take honors and advanced placement courses.
- Teacher expectations, i.e. the extent teachers expect students to

achieve at higher levels.
- The achievement gap, i.e. the difference in academic achievement between the average White student and the average Black and/or Latino student.
- The extent to which students can participate in classroom discussions, as well as how easily they can choose electives.
- The prevalence of suspensions, fights, drugs, alcohol, and gang-related behavior.

Jeynes' results revealed that religious school students generally outperform academically and behaviorally. Only one of the ninety studies showed faith-based schools underperforming. This is consistent with a Thomas Fordham Institute study of Catholic schools, which determined such students show more self-control and self-discipline than those in public schools as well as in other private schools.[22] The findings are particularly noteworthy given that religious schools spend far less money per student than public schools. "Educational efficiency, which focuses on how well school and government officials spend money, may be more important than how much is spent," writes Jeynes.[23]

As for charter schools, those students didn't outperform public school students; their results were about the same. Fifty-three percent of the studies indicated charter schools underperform public schools.

Two reasons why religious schools outperform, writes Jeynes, is they encourage more students to be on the academic (i.e. college) track, and parents are more involved. He observes that teachers at faith-based schools tend to be more demanding, and expect more rigorous courses and higher academic achievement regardless of socioeconomic status. Moreover the achievement gap is smaller. Jeynes suggests a possible reason for this is "religious educators are more likely to believe that children, no matter what their color and background, can achieve and reach great potential."

He cited another scholar who suggested African Americans perform better academically in faith-based schools because those schools "are more likely to see people as equal because they are made in the image of God" and thus demand high standards for everyone. Other scholars point to an ethic of working hard as a means of fulfilling a heavenly calling. The cumulative result is greater social capital among religious school students.

Meanwhile, public schools outperformed religious schools in classroom flexibility. Those students reported having greater opportunities to participate in classroom discussions as well as to choose electives. "By their sheer enrollment advantage and employment base, it seems intuitive that public schools might possess a greater inherent ability to offer a wider array of classes to their students." Jeynes says religious schools have emphasized the basics, with fewer electives.[24]

Onward to College

It's time to put to rest the misconception that more religious people are less educated. That may have been the case in times past, but not anymore. "While being raised in no religious tradition was once predictive of higher odds of completing a college degree, the trend has reversed," writes Horwitz. "For individuals born after 1960, being raised in no religious tradition is associated with lower odds of completing a 4-year college degree."[25] In another paper, she along with two other colleagues observe, "More religious adolescents are more interested in going to college."[26]

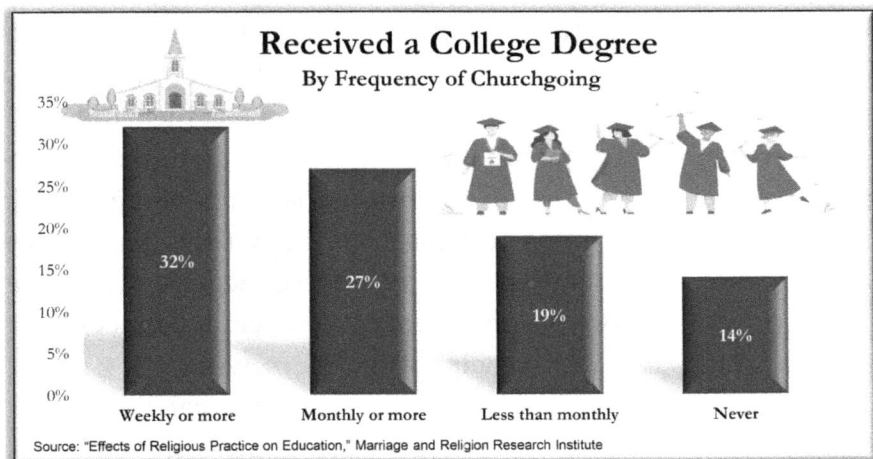

Received a College Degree
By Frequency of Churchgoing

Weekly or more	Monthly or more	Less than monthly	Never
32%	27%	19%	14%

Source: "Effects of Religious Practice on Education," Marriage and Religion Research Institute

Just as with completing high school, the more often a youth goes to church the likelier he or she is to complete college. Patrick Fagan of the Marriage and Religion Research Institute analyzed the National Survey of Family Growth, finding that 14 percent of never-churchgoers hold a bachelor's degree, versus 32 percent of weekly attenders.[27]

Churchgoing encourages marriage and marriage stability, which in turn encourages educational attainment. In analyzing the American Community Survey and the National Longitudinal Survey of Youth, a team lead by Brad Wilcox confirmed that compared with those who grew up with a single parent or in a stepfamily, young adults from intact families are much more likely to have a college degree.[28]

Regarding the college experience itself, four Texas State scholars led by William De Soto surprisingly found no association between religiosity and academic performance, honesty, or personal stress. However they did find a positive effect of religiosity on academic ethic. They distributed an 87-item questionnaire to undergraduates at a large, ethnically diverse southwestern university (probably Texas State, although they don't state the name). In addition to religiosity, the survey included questions about academic attitudes and performance, drinking and drugs, and various stressors they may face. As De Soto and colleagues describe it, to have a strong academic ethic is to be intrinsically motivated to learn and to regard one's classes as engaging. Such students take challenging courses because they like the process of learning. The scholars write, "This finding indicates that religious students tended to report being more engaged and devoted to their education than other students." Also of note, they ascertained that members of fraternities and sororities, as well as those living off campus, have a poorer academic ethic compared with other students. "Perhaps Greek life devalues academic pursuits," suggest De Soto and colleagues. "Religious groups provide a more positive form of social capital that encourages students to care about their college coursework."[29]

They list key points of various other studies comparing religious with nonreligious students. The results sometimes conflict, but religious students have the upper hand most of the time. Among the conclusions of the disparate studies, religious students:

- have modestly more academic success, although some evangelical students' time spent on spiritual activities caused their studying time to suffer.
- are less likely to drink alcohol to excess, but they didn't appear less likely to abuse prescription drugs.
- who regularly attended church as high school seniors had higher GPAs during college.
- don't necessarily have higher GPAs. (Those who conducted this study attributed the finding "to the limited and possibly unrepresentative nature of their survey data.")
- cope better with stress.
- have a higher level of personal distress.
- show no difference in depressive symptoms.
- show a negative correlation between emotional health and participation in campus religious groups.
- have higher levels of stress and anxiety (based on a small sample of students at a small university in the Southwest).
- are more satisfied at college and with their college experience.
- have greater equanimity.
- have a heightened sense of control over their life and surroundings.
- have a poorer academic ethic. (This was from a survey of fundamentalist Christians, whereas De Soto et al. polled religiously affiliated students in general.)

Meanwhile, another recent study of 775 students at public and private colleges in the U.S. Southwest estimated the following:

- attending church more than once a week: 75 percent lower likelihood of depression.
- praying daily: 60-70 percent lower likelihood of depression.
- intrinsic (very devout) religiosity: 51-69 percent lower likelihood.

The investigators observe, "Inclusion of religiosity/spirituality-oriented strategies may be important for mental health interventions in emerging adulthood."[30]

That's good advice, considering that college and university students are in the midst of a full-blown mental-health crisis. Based on 2019 statistics, an unbelievable 45 percent of them "felt so depressed that it was difficult to function" at least once during the year prior to being surveyed—up from 30 percent in 2011. Two out of three or 66 percent "felt overwhelming anxiety" and 43 percent "felt overwhelming anger." Equally alarming, more than one in ten college students—13 percent—seriously considered suicide.[31] And that was pre-Covid.

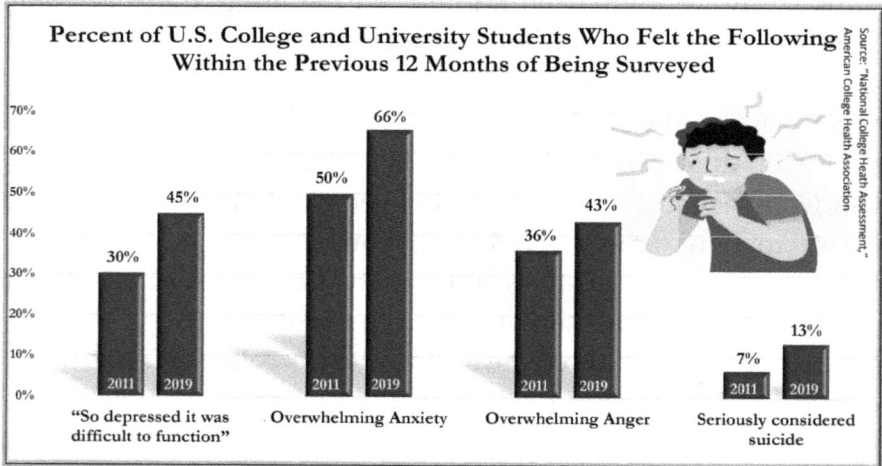

Percent of U.S. College and University Students Who Felt the Following Within the Previous 12 Months of Being Surveyed

Source: "National College Heath Assessment," American College Health Association

A college-student-oriented publication reporting some of these statistics offers several recommendations to address the crisis. In yet another sign of the ironies of our times, there's no mention of church and prayer.[32]

Sanctifying Sports

"I don't think I could do anything without the Lord in my life. He has been the one that has guided me, the one that has protected me, the one that has healed me when I had all those torn hamstrings and was frustrated, didn't know whether I wanted to continue to compete in track and field. So He kept me I'd say faithful. It was a lot of hard work, but I stayed faithful and stuck to it, and National Champion."[33]

So said a star athlete when reflecting on God playing a significant role. As discussed in chapters 6 and 7, religion can boost motivation to achieve goals by giving them a sacred significance, or sanctification. Even ordinary or mundane things can take on transcendent characteristics. And when it comes to larger endeavors, the greater the sanctification the greater the commitment to excel. When an activity is considered to be imbued with sacred qualities, it boosts confidence in one's ability to carry it out. That certainly includes sports.

Substantial numbers of athletes consider their sports involvement as sacred to some extent. Quinten K. Lynn wrote his Ph.D. dissertation at Bowling Green State on the extent to which athletes consider participation in their sport as having religious significance. Drawing from a survey of seventy Division 1 collegiate male and female athletes from a Midwestern university (he doesn't say which) covering sixteen sports, Lynn found that sports sanctification was not uncommon. Almost a third of respondents strongly agreed with the statement "God played a role in my sport career." More than half agreed with, "My participation in sport is part of a larger spiritual plan." Seeing sacredness in one's sport can only be a good thing as far as excelling in it. Such athletes are more likely to invest in and dedicate themselves to their endeavor, in addition to boosting confidence.

It's important to be able to cope with the highs and lows associated with being a serious athlete, be it losses and wins, coach-player interaction, injuries, or demanding schedules. Religion is a big help; athletes draw upon their beliefs to deal with the challenges. To be sure, none of the athletes in Lynn's study said they prayed to win. Instead, they considered the outcome of the competition and/or their ability to perform to be according to God's will. And they prayed to help them deal with stress. Or they prayed for the safety of themselves, teammates, and opponents. They gave thanks for their athletic abilities and for the opportunity to compete. "When I would step onto the field, I would basically say, okay, God, I am thankful for my family. And through my intensity on the field today, I am going to show you how thankful I am. I would use this as a form of motivation," related an athlete.[34]

Through losses, injury, difficult personalities, and other stressful factors, athletes are vulnerable to getting depressed now and again. Can religion help protect against this? Lynn cites a study concluding that in sports as in other walks of life, religiousness acts as a buffer against the blues—and against substance abuse. Despite strict rules forbidding it, high school and college athletes can be notorious for drinking and perhaps to a lesser extent, drugs. Lynn cites another study finding that greater religiosity and sports-sanctification are associated with less marijuana and alcohol consumption.

Commented Lynn, "Spirituality, it appears, is not checked in the locker room or left on the bench before athletes enter the game... For many student athletes, their involvement in sport is more than recreation, physical activity, or a quest for achieving lofty goals. It represents a sacred experience, an experience wherein they commune with the holy. As one athlete put it, 'My sport is a type of meditation for me...a time to grow closer with God.'"[35]

Shunning Drugs and Alcohol

As with athletes, among teens in general an anti-drug attitude is stronger among regular churchgoers, who also tend to avoid having drug-using friends. Religious teens are significantly less likely to abuse alcohol or smoke marijuana and cigarettes, according to a study published in *Psychology of Addictive Behaviors*.[36] (The study was done before the rise of vaping, which no doubt can be added to the list.) Another study found that just 10 percent of churchgoing girls between ages nine and seventeen reported using drugs or alcohol, versus 38 percent of all those surveyed.[37] And among high schoolers, according to a Texas A&M/Indiana University investigative team, religiosity delays alcohol consumption by three years.[38]

Jason Fletcher and Sanjeev Kumar of the Yale School of Public Health analyzed the Add Health survey, looking at the correlation between religiosity and legal and illegal substances. Self-reported importance of religion during adolescence "has the most significant effects on reducing dependence on use and abuse of addictive substances."[39] Another study found that among both married and single parents, church attendance and other religious activities with 12-14 year-olds were directly tied to less delinquent behavior two years later.[40]

Dads, embrace faith. It will help keep your kids away from drugs and booze. Drug addicts' fathers tend to have low levels of religiosity—even when the mother is religiously involved. And alcoholics with religious backgrounds tend to have strongly religious mothers but only moderately or nonreligious fathers. Also, if the religious beliefs of one parent significantly differ from those of the other, their child is more likely to abuse alcohol compared with children of parents with similar religious beliefs.[41]

Chapter 9

CHURCH AND SEX

A thirty-something year-old woman once related that after high school, she went overseas as an exchange student. "During that year abroad, I was very promiscuous. But the fact is, it cost me to be separated from myself. The longest-standing wound I gave myself was heartfelt. That sick, used feeling of having given a precious part of myself—my soul—to so many and for nothing, still aches. I never imagined I'd pay so dearly and for so long…Sex without commitment is very risky for the heart."[1]

Hers is an all-too common story. With feelings of guilt, remorse, self-contempt, and shame, the emotional toll of premarital sex often lasts years, sometimes a lifetime. Whereas about 7 percent of teenage non-sexually active girls report being depressed, it's 25 percent for sexually active ones. For boys the numbers are 3.5 percent and 8 percent respectively.[2] That seems on the low side for boys, but plenty of them have regrets: 53 percent wish they would have waited. For girls it's 67 percent.[3]

Those numbers no doubt persist into adulthood. Not only does depression set in, but lives get derailed. One college student was so distraught over a failed sexual relationship that he dropped out of college. He recounted, "I couldn't keep my mind on my studies. I just wanted to lie down and die. Finally, I knew I was flunking out, so I quit college and joined the Navy"[4] (which, of course, also is a very admirable life choice).

Another young man stuck with college but wasn't happy. "…A few days later, we broke up. It was the most painful time of my life. I had opened up to her more than anybody, even my parents.

I was depressed and nervous. I dropped out of sports and felt like a failure. In college, I've had mostly one-night stands. I'm afraid of falling in love."[5]

Teen girls who had sex were six times more likely to commit suicide than girls who had not.[6] The study was from 1991 but it's a sure bet the story is similar today.

"I don't think I ever met a student who was sorry he or she had postponed sexual activity, but I certainly met many who deeply regretted their sexual involvements," related a former English professor in an email to psychologist and educator Thomas Lickona. "No one prepares young people for the after-effects: the lowered self-esteem; the despairing sense of having been used; the self-contempt for being a user…"[7]

Churchgoers, of course, are much less likely to have premarital sex. Same with abortion, where the consequences can rear their ugly heads years later. A mother in her thirties reflected on the abortion she had in college. "If someone had asked me right then how I felt about what I had just done, I would have said, 'Wow, this is great! I have my health back, I have my life back!'" Then her tone shifted. "Go ahead, ask me now. I am, at this moment, crying."[8]

The website afterabortion.com helps women heal after that event. As reported by Miriam Grossman, a former campus psychiatrist at UCLA, a support board on the website listed titles of threads painting a heart-rending picture of what many women go through. "Need help—NOW!"; "I'm losing it…"; "Suffocating"; "Can't breathe"; "Tears won't stop"; "Oh man can it get any worse?"; "Sad Scared Alone"; "Breakdown"; "Someone please please help"; "Numb"; "Why??????????"; "Can't do this anymore."[9]

A meta-analysis covering more than 875,000 women found that having an abortion prompts an 81 percent higher risk of mental health problems compared with women who carry their unintended pregnancy to term. The problems include depression, anxiety, drug and alcohol abuse, and suicidal behaviors, according to Priscilla Coleman of Bowling Green State, publishing her results in *The British Journal of Psychiatry*.[10] And it's not just women who are hurting.

In a *Los Angeles Times* poll, more than two-thirds of men whose girlfriends or wives had an abortion indicated they experienced guilt. A third of them felt regret.[11]

Beware the Health Hazards

Piled onto the long-term emotional consequences of premarital sex are physical perils. There are at least twenty-five types of sexually transmitted diseases. Four common STDs are chlamydia, gonorrhea, syphilis, and trichomoniasis. Long-term effects may include itching and burning in the genital region and elsewhere, chronic pain, sterility and infertility, throat infections, pelvic inflammatory disease (PID), cancer, immune system disorders, and sometimes even death. Diseases and symptoms can be passed from mothers to babies. In some cases STDs are harder to treat now because of immunity to antibiotics.[12]

An earlier age for first-time sex boosts the risks of STDs and of course pregnancy. Teenage sex augments the likelihood of other risky activities including drinking, smoking, and substance abuse.[13] Those who choose abortion not only end a life but also increase the risk of breast cancer later in life by an estimated 30 percent. In addition to the above-mentioned emotional consequences, abortion also is linked to cervical cancer, ovarian cancer, infertility, and PID.[14]

As Grossman writes, "The message must get out: casual sex is a health hazard for young women." She affirmed the only way to avoid its mental and physical consequences is for both women and men to wait until marriage—and once married, remain faithful.[15] Those most likely to fit this description go to church regularly and take their faith very seriously.

Weakening the Marriage Bond

The emotional and physical fallout takes its toll in the marriage sphere. An active sexual history can make it harder to find a spouse and, once found, can evoke guilt and regret. Sexual relations create a hormonal bonding between individuals. As those bonds are continually broken with multiple sex partners, the ability to properly connect with that special someone weakens.[16] "Sexual flashbacks" of previous partners can disrupt intimacy with a spouse. The chances of adultery are higher, as those with many previous flings may find it harder to resist temptation.

Love affairs with sexual pleasures early on end up being more fragile in the long run and may undermine other aspects of relationship development. For example, with sex at the forefront the couple may not put as much energy into communication. And becoming prematurely enmeshed in sex may prompt a person to stay with someone with whom he or she otherwise would break up due to incompatibility issues, resulting in a more brittle marriage. This "relationship inertia" particularly can be a factor when a couple cohabits.

The preceding points are based on a study by Dean Busby, Jason Carroll, and Brian Willoughby of BYU who analyzed a survey of 2,035 married individuals regarding when they first became sexually involved, and the current state of their marriage and overall well-being. The undeniable conclusion is that couples who save sex for marriage are likelier to be happier and more stable. Relationship satisfaction is 20 percent higher and relationship stability 22 percent higher. The icing on the cake? Sexual quality is 15 percent higher. "It is clear that the longer a couple waited to become sexually involved the better their sexual quality, relationship communication, relationship satisfaction, and perceived relationship stability was in marriage," write the investigators.[17]

University of Utah's Nicholas Wolfinger echoed the above findings in his study on marital happiness as it relates to sexual history. Men who just had one partner in their lifetime are more likely to have "very happy" marriages. Sixty-five percent of women who only had sexual relations with their husbands reported being very happy in their marriage. For married women who had six to ten previous relationships where things got physical, the number drops to 52 percent very happy. Most of the women in the one-partner category—almost 70 percent—were churchgoers. Only about 30 percent of those who had ten or more sexual sweethearts reported being churchgoers.[18]

Regardless of whether a person engaged in premarital sex, simply having beliefs and attitudes approving of uncommitted sex can negatively impact the marital relationship. Juliana French and two other Florida State professors of psychology confirmed this after surveying more than 200 newly married couples over the course of a few years, and determining which ones had filed for divorce. Couples in which both spouses generally believe uncommitted sex is okay suffered lower relationship satisfaction over time, and more divorce. They reported "lower commitment, fewer relationship-maintenance motivations, decreased sexual interest in their partners, increased attention to attractive extra-pair partners, and more frequent infidelity," wrote the investigators. "Unrestricted sociosexuality may undermine processes inherent to long-term relationship maintenance that negatively impact intimates' relationship satisfaction and long-term stability."[19]

Even if the marital relationship is strong, sexual history can come back to haunt. Countless women are infertile because of an STD from years earlier. Said a thirty-three-year-old wife, "Sometime during my wild college days, I picked up an infection that damaged the inside of my fallopian tubes and left me infertile. I am now married to a wonderful man who very much wants children, and the guilt I feel is overwhelming. We will look into adoption, but this whole ordeal has been terribly difficult."[20]

Faith Cultivates Chastity

Whereas popular culture encourages premarital sex by trumpeting pleasure and instant gratification, religion discourages it by emphasizing scripture teachings and delayed gratification. Stronger faith, more frequent prayers, and greater church attendance are associated with a longer duration of abstinence. By and large, the more religious and churchgoing the person, the fewer sexual partners and the later age of first-time sex. A study found that 48 percent of teen girls who had not yet had sex cited religious and/ or moral reasons.[21]

Religiosity is associated with delayed first sex not only directly in the sense of refusal to violate religious teachings but indirectly based on fear of emotional distress, which may in turn stem from religious upbringing. Prudent teens don't want to deal with guilt, embarrassment of pregnancy and/or of STDs, loss of respect from a love interest, and/or upsetting one's parents. Ann Meier of UW-Madison analyzed data from the Add Health survey, selecting 5,000 youth ages 15 to 18. Her findings indicate religiosity significantly reduces the likelihood of teen girls having sex in the following year, and to a lesser extent lowered the likelihood of teen boys doing so.[22]

More religious families are associated with less adolescent sex because the parents tend to spend more time around their children, and monitor them and who their friends are to a greater extent, according to Jennifer Manlove and colleagues at Child Trends. Such children also may have more religiously inclined friends, generating further moral pressure against sex. Studies show that compared with non-sexually active teens, sexually active ones tend to participate less in family activities, undergo less monitoring by parents, and have lower-quality relationships with parents.[23]

Pledging Abstinence

Society and the media are replete with messages that make nonmarital sex appear appealing and normal. Kids and adults alike are bombarded with words, images, songs, videos, social media, websites, movies, TV shows, magazines, and other influences that encourage it. That makes it all the more difficult to resist. "Remaining abstinent or making responsible sexual decisions during the adolescent years may be one of the most significant challenges facing youth today," commented Lynn Blinn-Pike of the University of Missouri's Center on Adolescent Sexuality, Pregnancy and Parenting. "The number of sexual messages that adolescents receive via the print and mass media each day makes it a challenging circumstance to be sexually resilient." She calls such resistance sexual resiliency.

Writing in 1999, she pointed to the societal transformation that occurred from the 1960s to 1990s. During the sixties, common topics on television included dates, jobs, and cars. By the 1990s they included pregnancy, sexual abuse, STDs, sexual harassment, and suicide. She reported that based on a study conducted in the late 1980s, on daytime television dramas the ratio of unmarried to married partners was 24 to 1, sending the message that sex typically occurs outside of marriage.[24]

How can a teen stand a chance in such a sex-crazed world? Despite the debauchery, or perhaps because of it, in the 1990s public "virginity pledges" came onto the scene. Youth promised to avoid sex until marriage.

Do virginity pledges work? Despite portrayals in the media misleading people into thinking they don't, it has been confirmed that for many youths, they do. Jeremy Uecker of the sociology department at UT Austin found that pledgers as well as churchgoers are still much more likely to remain virgins until marriage than non-pledgers and non-churchgoers. And when they do have premarital relations, pledgers are more likely to do so only with their future spouse. "Religion and abstinence pledging are powerful and robust predictors of abstinence until marriage and limiting premarital sex to only a future spouse, at least among Americans who marry at a relatively young age," he writes.

Peter Bearman and Hannah Brückner of Columbia University echo those findings, concluding that those who signed a pledge were much less likely than non-pledgers to lose their virginity a year later. They estimate that pledgers' relative risk of sexual initiation is 34 percent lower than non-pledgers. However, an interesting dynamic is that in schools in which the students form the vast majority of their friendships and romantic relationships with fellow schoolmates (as opposed to schools where many friendships are with kids from other schools), if too many students in a school take the pledge—more than around 30 percent of the student body—the pledge doesn't have a significant effect on preventing premarital sex. This is because youth view it as an identity movement; when everyone is pledging, it seems to lose its specialness or uniqueness. The authors note that this is a common phenomenon with identity movements. Also of note, in schools where many friendships are with kids from other schools, when there are no other pledgers in that school, virginity pledging has little or no effect.[25]

Those who took the True Love Waits pledge delayed premarital sex by eighteen months on average, according to one study. And there's a subgroup that stands out: the 16 percent of American teenagers who rate religion as being "extremely important" to them. "When these guys pledge, they mean it," writes Hanna Rosin in *Slate*. She spent a year among such teens and can attest to their strong self-discipline in refraining from sex. "They can spend all evening sitting on the couch holding hands and nothing more. They can date for a year, be alone numerous times in a car or at the movies, and still stick to what's known in the Christian youth literature as 'side hugs,' to avoid excessive touching," she recounts.[26]

For abstinence pledgers and religious Americans who aren't so disciplined, premarital sex is still widespread. This is no surprise; it can be hard to stay chaste living in a society where sexual temptations and permissiveness abound. Uecker writes, "Even the most religious individuals will not be entirely isolated from secular messages about sex, and when religious sexual scripts are forced to compete against less restrictive ones (in addition to biological impulses), they seem to lose out most of the time. It could be argued that this prevalence of premarital sex is a sign of the diminished influence of institutional religion on sexual behavior, and this very well may be the case."

On the brighter side, Uecker observes that "Remarkably, married young adults who attended religious services weekly or more during adolescence are nearly eight times more likely to abstain from sex until marriage than those who never attended. There is also a marked difference between regular and semi-regular attenders: Only 8 percent of the semi-regulars wait until marriage to have sex, compared to 21 percent of regular attenders." Likewise, 8 percent of those who don't take the virginity pledge delay sex until marriage, versus 27 percent of pledgers. And 59 percent of pledgers only have premarital sex with their future spouse.[27]

Mormons Most Chaste

Upon analyzing Add Health, Uecker saw that Mormons are the most likely to abstain from sex until marriage, with an abstinence rate of about 43 percent—versus 3 percent for nonreligious. Mormon youth as a whole are much more chaste than conservative/evangelical Protestants, who have a 15 percent abstinence rate. The rates for mainline Protestants, Catholics, and Black Protestants are 10 percent, 9 percent, and 5 percent respectively. Even though Blacks have a relatively high rate of religiosity, Uecker reports that throughout the history of the Black Protestant church, clergy generally have been reluctant to discuss sexual issues. "As a result, any religious teachings against premarital sex may be quickly drowned out by other, more sexually permissive messages in secular culture." A similar phenomenon holds true for Catholics, who "may not be particularly effective in socializing their young adults' sexual behavior." That's painfully ironic because Catholic teaching holds that premarital sex is a mortal sin—i.e. it lands you in hell, assuming you don't confess it to a priest during the sacrament of confession. Just a small percentage of Catholics even regularly go to confession. Among Catholic bishops, priests, youth ministers, and educators, dereliction of duty abounds.

What accounts for Mormons' relative wholesomeness? Uecker observes that they attend regular religious education classes known as seminary—typically for ages 14 through 18—which include plentiful teachings on sexual ethics. Participants in Mormon temple rituals are often required to be sexually chaste. They take virginity pledges at a higher rate than other denominations with the exception of conservative/evangelical Protestants. Mormons' spurning of alcohol reduces their exposure to situations conducive to sexual activity. And whether it be Mormon or another denomination or religion, it's the teachings of the religion itself that strongly deter premarital sex—even more so than warnings about STDs and unwanted pregnancy, according to Uecker.[28]

The last point is consistent with a New Zealand study finding that it's mainly religious teachings and not secular teachings of morality that influence whether students engage in sex. "There were few socioeconomic, family, or individual factors that distinguished those who had had intercourse from those who had not by age 21," wrote the study authors. The main factor was religion: "Persistent religious involvement showed the strongest relationship with abstinence."[29]

Another study drew a somewhat different conclusion—that the most common reason for avoiding teen sex is fear of pregnancy and/or STDs, with the second-most common reason religious beliefs. That's according to Blinn-Pike's survey of 697 eighth- through tenth graders. (The least-common reason is cost and availability of birth control.)[30] Ironically, in some instances religiosity can increase the likelihood of pregnancy and STDs; religious individuals who do become sexually active tend to use contraception less, perhaps thinking they'll never engage in sex but in the heat of passion decide otherwise.

Among Muslims as well, higher religiosity is protective against premarital sex, as Islam prohibits it. A study analyzed a U.S. national college survey of 10,401 students, of whom 1.3 percent or 135 indicated they were raised in Muslim families. It determined that for the unmarried among them, 57 percent of males and 48 percent of females had ever had sex—which are relatively low numbers amid a secular society in which pressures for premarital sex are legion.[31]

Chapter 10

STAVING OFF SUICIDE

In the 2005 movie *Constantine*, Keanu Reeves plays John Constantine, an exorcist who can see angels and demons. His soul is destined for hell for the mortal sin of suicide; when he was a teenager he attempted to take his own life but was revived—after spending two minutes in hell. Rachel Weisz plays a detective whose twin sister committed suicide. She seeks out the assistance of Constantine, who confirms her sister's soul is in hell.

The movie reinforces Christian—especially Catholic—notions of suicide: that it's a one-way ticket to hell. (According to Catholic teachings, exceptions can be made for grave psychological disturbances, in which case a soul could land in purgatory instead, the lowest level of which is said to be similar to hell in terms of the suffering, but not eternal.) Judaism and Islam also prohibit suicide, and Hinduism and Buddhism strongly discourage it.

The hell factor is a powerful deterrent. Noelle Garcia, Catholic speaker and recording artist, in an audio presentation discussed her psychological struggles as a teenager, obsessing about jealousy, looks, popularity, and the like. She started cutting herself in an effort to relieve emotional pain. "The only thing that saved my life was that I believed if I killed myself I would go to hell, and I didn't want to go to hell. I believed in the existence of hell. I thought about suicide all the time," she related.[1]

Fear of hell no doubt helps explain why the suicide rate among the devoutly religious is far lower than among the nonreligious. In fact, among Christians who do take their own lives, surely the vast majority of them either didn't attend church or attended one where the minister or priest avoids the topic of hell and/or adopts the attitude that everyone goes to heaven (which, even though it's contrary to biblical teaching, probably is the majority sentiment these days). Suicide victims who truly believed in hell and its eternal agonies, and who truly believed suicide triggers automatic damnation, must account for a tiny percentage of suicide cases; perhaps for some reason they thought they deserved hell.

Christianity considers suicide a grave sin that violates the commandment "Thou shalt not kill." New York Department of Transportation worker Isidor "Izzy" Suarez once talked someone out of jumping off a bridge. He asked him if he was Christian, to which the hapless man replied in the affirmative. "If you kill yourself, it's like murder," warned Suarez. In other words, killing yourself is as serious a sin as killing someone else. After ruminating over Suarez's admonishment, the man abandoned the attempt on his life.[2]

It isn't just the threat of hell that deters suicide. It's the incentive of heaven, along with hope and meaning. Melodie, an Asian-American college student and accomplished tennis player, said that if it weren't for Jesus, she wouldn't be here. Her religious beliefs prevented her from jumping off a building. "The presence or lack of hope can mean the difference between life and death," writes Miriam Grossman. "Melodie draws hope from Psalms and the Gospel of Luke. She carried a Bible in her backpack. Sometimes she prays between classes."[3]

With heaven and hope in mind, you can more readily endure the trials of life, be it sickness or injury, job loss, the death of a loved one, or financial hardships. Role models in the Bible include Job, who endured great suffering yet still valued life and loved God, with no thought of taking his own life (though he cursed the day he was born). Suffering can be accepted as God's plan, as penance for sins, or as an opportunity to grow in character. Religion can prompt you to focus on getting ahead spiritually rather than through wealth, status, or other worldly values. "A quest for spiritual success may replace the quest for material success," writes Steven Stack of Penn State's sociology department. Stack also notes that a war mentality against Satan can arouse passions and eliminate any thought of suicide.[4]

Francie Hart Broghammer, the chief psychiatry resident at UC Irvine Medical Center, says religious faith can instill meaning and purpose, helping to quell anguish and turn suffering into something meaningful. "I have seen this first-hand, time and time again," she recounted, "with many of my patients reporting they would have attempted suicide long ago if they did not have faith, which provided them with hope in otherwise hopeless circumstances."[5]

Of course, atheism or agnosticism don't cause suicide—there are plenty of happy nonbelievers who would never dream of such an act. And when the going gets tough, there's still a lot of social, familial, and moral pressure to refrain from taking their lives. But sometimes that isn't enough. The absence of another key safeguard can push them over the edge. It may be what happened to Jesse Kilgore.[6] Not only did Richard Dawkins' *The God Delusion* possibly help remove from this impressionable young man that key safeguard against suicide—religion—but it may have helped quash in him a sense of meaning and purpose. Atheism assumes only the physical world exists, and that physical particles illogically came into existence on their own. Equally illogically, the vast array of particles, components, and subcomponents somehow spontaneously assembled themselves into wondrously engineered cells and living beings by random chance with zero planning or purpose and zero input from an intelligent Creator. To atheists, we're just bodies and no soul. As Dawkins bleakly remarked, "You are for nothing. You are here to propagate your selfish genes. There is no higher purpose in life."[7] Another observer put it more colorfully. We're nothing more than "the forward edge of the sludge of evolution."[8] Being under the false impression that this is all we are, why go on living? Jesse Kilgore took that to heart.

It's a shame Kilgore abandoned his faith. He was one of the many victims of deaths of despair that have become so common of late, especially amid pandemic-induced social isolation. Even prior to the Covid lockdowns, suicide was the second-leading cause of death among U.S. adolescents and tenth-leading cause among adults.[9] It's no surprise that suicide has been rising while churchgoing has been falling. In 2004 only 44 percent of Americans reported they had attended church or synagogue in the last seven days. In 2020 it was down to an abysmal 30 percent.[10] During that time suicide increased by more than 25 percent in the United States—again, even before Covid (updated statistics aren't available as of this writing).[11]

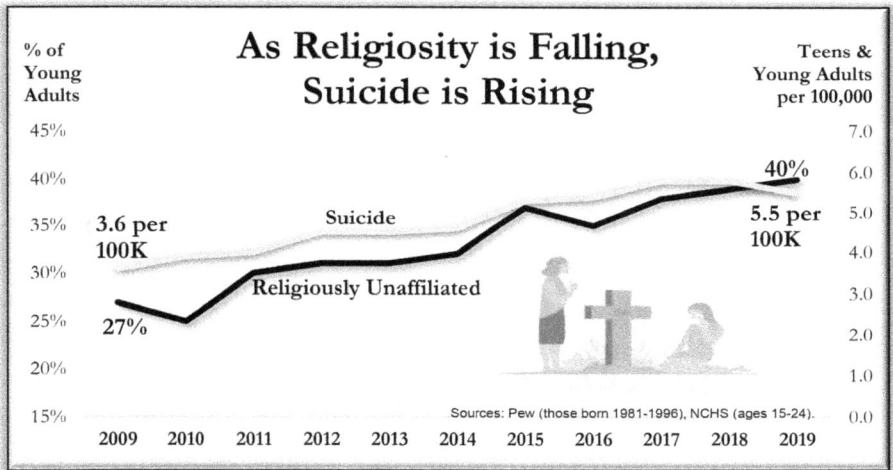

With suicide reaching epidemic proportions, people should be shouting from the rooftops to get back to church. It's the single most effective weapon against self-harm. In 2016, Harvard epidemiologists Tyler VanderWeele, Shanshan Li, and Ichiro Kawachi reported Center for Disease Control statistics showing that from 1999 to 2014, suicides increased from 10.5 to 13.0 per 100,000 people. During that period, based on Gallup polling data, weekly church attendance declined from 43 percent of the U.S. population to 36 percent. The scholars declared, "If we were to extrapolate our study estimate to the general population, this would indicate that *nearly 40% of the increase in the suicide rate could be attributed to the decline in religious service attendance.*"[12] (emphasis added)

VanderWeele also confirmed that 40 percent of the increase in mental illness in recent decades stems from the decline in religious service attendance.[13]

Evidence that churchgoing combats suicide is legion:

- Frequent churchgoers are four times less likely to take their own lives than never-attenders.[14]

- Among older Americans, those who neglect church have 4.34 higher odds of committing suicide than regular attenders.[15]

- Of the 70 studies Objective Hope reviewed examining the effect of religiosity on preventing suicide, 61 found a positive effect, eight no effect, one mixed, and none found a negative effect.

- Of 141 studies Koenig and colleagues surveyed on the subject, 106 found religion is associated with fewer suicides or suicide attempts, less suicide ideation, and/or negative attitudes towards suicide.[16]

People showing up at church at least two-dozen times a year are less than half as likely to kill themselves than those going less often, according to George Mason University's Evan Kleinman and Brown University's Richard Liu. They write, "Frequent attendance at religious services may be an indicator of consistent exposure to others who provide social support. It may also be an indicator of how much one adheres to the tenets of one's religion, including internalizing anti-suicidal beliefs...The current findings are consistent with Joiner's interpersonal theory of suicide, which posits that having a sense of belonging is negatively associated with suicidal desire."[17]

It had been thought the unemployment rate was the biggest predictor of suicide. It turns out that isn't necessarily the case. Church attendance likely is more significant. While unemployment can lead to depression and then suicide, that's much less likely to happen to an unemployed person who regularly attends church. According to Stack, "The findings on unemployment indicate that once a control is introduced for the religious factor, the unemployment-suicide relationship is often greatly reduced...While both variables are often significant, the religious factor is generally more closely associated with the variance in suicide."[18]

In addition to reasons discussed above, less suicide among the religiously devout stems from teachings that:

- prohibit or discourage alcohol or excessive amounts of it, as its abuse can lead to depression and suicide.

- disallow marijuana and other street drugs.

- forbid extramarital sex and sexual promiscuity, which could lead to relationship complexities and resulting mental turmoil.

- facilitate and encourage strong social and family ties, reducing social isolation. Not only do religions emphasize the importance of family, but they provide venues to meet and spend time with like-minded people, building friendships.

- emphasize the sanctity of life, which discourages depressed or infirm persons from taking their lives.

Some of the above factors are reflected in a study on depressed inpatients carried out by a Columbia University team led by Kanita Dervic. Evaluated were 371 patients at the New York State Psychiatric Institute as well as at the Western Psychiatric Institute and Clinic in Pittsburgh. Dervic and the team compared religiously affiliated with religiously unaffiliated patients. Averaged out, each group was the same in terms of education, income, gender, and race. The religiously unaffiliated were about five years younger on average (33 versus 37), were single to a greater extent, and less often had children. They also had more nonfamilial relationships (friends and acquaintances) whereas the religiously affiliated on average had a more family-oriented social network. Observe Dervic and colleagues, "We found weaker family ties in religiously unaffiliated subjects, and family members are reported to be more likely to provide reliable emotional support, nurturance, and reassurance of worth. Our finding is consistent with reports about less dense social networks among atheists." They note that the greatest protective effect of religion on suicide is among those who have relatives and friends who share their religion.

The religiously unaffiliated had significantly higher lifetime scores for substance abuse, aggression, and impulsivity, but not for hostility. They reported fewer reasons for living, based on factors that include a weaker sense of responsibility toward one's family and a lower moral objection to suicide. They also were more likely to have had first-degree relatives who ended their lives. Not surprisingly, the unaffiliated had the highest number of attempts. And past attempts are the best predictor of future suicide or attempts.

The religiously unaffiliated and affiliated were, on average, the same in terms of level of depression. This suggests positive aspects of religiosity outweigh negative effects of depression and stressful life events. Moreover among depressed religious persons there's a higher threshold for suicidal thoughts. "Religion may provide a positive force that counteracts suicidal ideation in the face of depression, hopelessness, and stressful events," writes the study team.

Dervic and colleagues offer recommendations for mental health professionals. For suicidal patients wavering on or ambivalent about their religion, therapists should gently discuss those beliefs, particularly the beliefs' moral objections to suicide. Despite psychiatrists being less religious than the general population, "support of the patient's spirituality has been deemed an ethical imperative, reflecting a physician's commitment to the patient's best interest." Such support "could be an additional resource in psychiatric and psychotherapeutic treatments targeting suicidal acts."[19]

Suicide Lower in More Religious Countries

Countries with low religiosity generally have higher suicide rates. Japan for example has one of the highest rates of atheism and agnosticism, and according to a Gallup poll one of the highest suicide rates. Other countries fitting that profile include Russia, Estonia, and Belgium. Conversely, countries with the highest levels of religiosity have the lowest suicide rates including Kuwait, the Philippines, and Paraguay. To be sure, correlation does not necessarily imply causation. Other factors could explain higher suicide rates. Perhaps it's weaker family ties, or greater use of technology (think Internet and social isolation). Gallup's Brett Pelham and Zsolt Nyiri observe that less-religious countries on the whole are wealthier yet suffer more suicide than more-religious countries. "The relation between

GDP and suicide is not nearly as strong as the relation between religiosity and suicide," they point out. "An analysis focusing only on wealthy countries, where documentation of suicide is likely to be excellent, still reveals a robust association between religiosity and (lower) national suicide rates."[20]

Catholic vs. Protestant

In one of the earliest empirical studies on suicide, in the late 1890s the eminent French sociologist Émile Durkheim (1858-1917) ascertained that in Europe, suicide rates were four times higher in Protestant countries and geographic regions compared with Catholic ones. That generally still holds true today—suicides are three times higher in Protestant regions according to a study analyzing Switzerland census data. Protestants have a lower suicide rate than the nonreligious, and Catholics a lower rate than Protestants. "The study suggests that Durkheim's observation persists, at least in Switzerland," writes VanderWeele.[21]

Durkheim argued that stronger social control and cohesion among Catholics explained the differing suicide rates. Out of concern for the negative effect of suicide on the larger community, a depressed Catholic is more reluctant to carry out such an act.[22]

The stronger cohesiveness stems from Catholics being bound by Vatican interpretation of the Bible, looking to official teachings of popes for guidance on how to live out biblical lessons. Protestantism, by contrast, prides itself on private interpretation of the Bible. It involves deducing meaning in sacred scriptures according to one's own predilections—or alternatively, relying on one's pastor or denomination for biblical interpretation. Individual autonomy is paramount. Some Protestants and/or Protestant denominations choose to observe strict rules in such areas as sexual ethics, modes and frequency of public worship, raising of children, etc., while other denominations are much more lax in those matters while believing in good conscience they're in conformance with the Bible.

Some of that now also applies within the Catholic Church. These days plenty of Catholics ignore many biblical teachings and seem not to care they're in violation thereof. And from parish to parish, certain teachings are elevated and certain ones downplayed depending on the theological leanings of the priest or bishop. So Durkheim's argument likely was stronger in his day, when Catholics generally were more devout and cohesive.

That's reflected in the work of economists Sascha Becker and Ludger Woessmann of the universities of Warwick and Munich respectively. They analyzed suicide data from nineteenth-century Prussia as well as twenty-first-century Europe, finding that the suicide rate among Prussian Protestants back then was about three times as high as among Catholics. According to their estimates, today it's about twice as high vis-à-vis majority Catholic countries versus majority Protestant ones.

Becker and Woessmann put forward another explanation for the differing suicide rates. In Catholic doctrine, good deeds are of paramount importance in gaining God's grace, while sin causes a loss of grace. Suicide is deemed a mortal sin, which sends a person to hell—or at least to a long and painful purgatory. By contrast, according to Protestant *sola gratia* (by grace alone) doctrine, God dispenses grace without regard to the merit of the person's deeds. Even with suicide, therefore, a person can avoid hell according to Protestants' belief—as well as purgatory since they don't believe in it. "This reasoning is consistent with the fact that, at least in modern Protestant doctrine, the predestination aspect leads to a more lenient assessment of suicide," write Becker and Woessmann.[23] (Note that with thousands of denominations of Protestantism, the preceding may not be true in all cases.)

Another deterrent to suicide within Catholicism is the sacrament of confession, in which Catholics orally confess their sins and especially mortal sins to a priest. Committing suicide obliterates any chance of confessing that sin, since the person is now dead. It's a strong disincentive to suicide. Among Protestants, confession isn't a sacrament and the doctrine of mortal sin is absent. When they do confess their sins, they typically do so mentally to God rather than through a third person. "Thus, both sociological and theological differences between Protestants and Catholics make suicide more likely among the former group," write the authors.[24]

In addition to the disincentive effect, lower suicide rates among Catholic countries likely stem from better mental health owing to confession. Being told by an authority that one's sins are forgiven is liberating, freeing one from guilt and anxiety. As philosopher and Lutheran theologian Paul Tillich wrote in 1948, "Mental diseases have become epidemic in the United States as well as in Europe. In this situation, psychoanalysis has seemed more desirable for educated people than religion, especially Protestant religion. In Catholic countries the situation has been different because the confession has been able to overcome many tendencies toward personal disintegration."[25]

Psychoanalyst Carl Jung (1875-1961) attributed the low level of neuroticism among Catholics to confession.[26] But that was prior to the Second Vatican Council (a.k.a. Vatican II) in the 1960s, which didn't change the core teachings of the Church but did change the culture of it. After that, most Catholics stopped going to confession. In the U.S. only about 15 percent of them do so at least several times a year, and almost half of Catholics never go.[27] Someone once said that prior to Vatican II, the fewest number of people in mental institutions were Catholics. After Vatican II, they were the most. If true, it would be no surprise.

(Devout) Catholics' Low Suicide Rate

In the wake of Vatican II, contrary to the teachings of their faith, many Catholic bishops and priests downplayed or rarely mentioned hell, purgatory, and mortal sin. That rubbed off on their congregations, no doubt resulting in more suicides among Catholics than would otherwise be the case. Fortunately there are still many Catholics who take the teachings seriously—so much so that they go to confession monthly or even weekly, and attend religious services (i.e. Catholic Mass) not just every Sunday but most every day. In fact, attending daily Mass reduces the likelihood to near zero that a person will ever commit suicide.

A Harvard study led by VanderWeele confirmed this. Of about 7,000 Catholic women who said they went to Mass more than once a week, not one committed suicide. It was data taken from the Nurses' Health Study, a long-term survey of tens of thousands of female nurses that began in 1976 and continues to the present day. The women were mainly Christians. Over the course of the study period there were thirty-six suicides (denoting a suicide rate among nurses to be about half the rate of U.S. women in general). Those attending religious services once a week or more were five times less likely to commit suicide than non-churchgoers. While Protestant regular churchgoers had a much lower likelihood of suicide than non-churchgoers including non-churchgoing Catholics, they still were seven times more likely to die by their own hand than devout Catholics.[28]

What is it about daily-Mass-going Catholics that so protects them from suicide? In addition to reasons discussed above—the concept of mortal sin, fear of hell, and the psychological benefits of confession—it simply could be the grace of God. The Catholic Church takes Jesus's words literally and not symbolically when in the Bible at the Last Supper he holds up the unleavened bread and wine and says "this is my body" and "this is my blood." (Matthew 26:26,28) At every Mass, the priest reenacts that on the altar. If the bread and wine truly become Christ's body and blood, then that goes a long way in explaining the effectiveness of this suicide prevention technique.

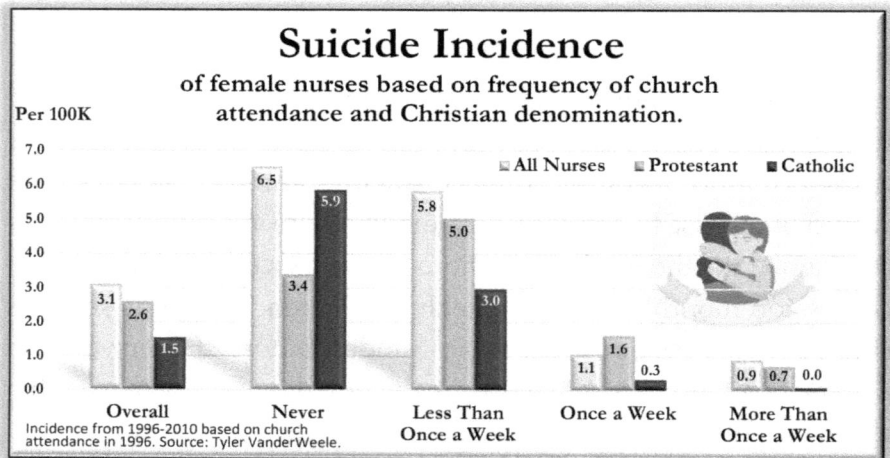

Suicide Incidence

of female nurses based on frequency of church attendance and Christian denomination.

Per 100K

☐ All Nurses ▨ Protestant ■ Catholic

	Overall	Never	Less Than Once a Week	Once a Week	More Than Once a Week
All Nurses	3.1	6.5	5.8	1.1	0.9
Protestant	2.6	3.4	5.0	1.6	0.7
Catholic	1.5	5.9	3.0	0.3	0.0

Incidence from 1996-2010 based on church attendance in 1996. Source: Tyler VanderWeele.

Other Faiths

Utah has one of the highest suicide rates in the nation. As the state has so many Mormons, that must mean there's something about the Mormon faith that leads adherents to suicide, right? Perhaps it stems from the church's strict demands and associated pressures on its members? Wrong. Just the opposite is the case. Young men active in the Mormon church in Utah are many times less likely to commit suicide than non-Mormons or Mormons who don't adhere to church doctrines and practices. Sterling Hilton, professor of statistics at BYU, along with other colleagues conducted a study confirming this. (It just focused on males aged 15-34.) "Many factors of religiosity relate to lowered suicide rates," Hilton told the BYU student newspaper *The Daily Universe*. "Latter-day Saints believe in a higher being, an afterlife, and the sanctity of life. They believe life, in and of itself, is precious. The church also has an elaborate social support system." One of its prohibitions is alcohol, which discourages suicide as alcohol abuse can be a factor in this tragic event. To be sure, the study found that Mormon males aged 25-34 who don't adhere to church doctrines and practices have a some- what higher suicide rate than non-Mormons in Utah.[29] This again shows the hazards of lukewarmness.

As noted above, other religions outlaw or discourage suicide to varying degrees. Jewish law forbids it; at least under Orthodox Judaism, persons who take their own lives may be buried in a sep- arate section of a Jewish cemetery, and possibly be denied certain mourning rites.[30]

Islam strictly forbids suicide; several passages in the Koran in- dicate hell awaits committers of this deed—and the method used will be imposed on them repeatedly for eternity. It's written in the Koran, "He who commits suicide by throttling shall keep on throttling himself in the Hell-Fire forever and he who commits suicide by stabbing himself shall keep on stabbing himself in the Hell-Fire." What about suicide bombings? Apparently there's a minority school of thought in Islam that in the case of jihad, the bomber isn't considered dead but living in paradise.[31]

While Hinduism isn't as forceful against suicide as Christianity, Judaism, and Islam, it strongly discourages it, considered to be on par with murder as it violates the code of *ahimsa* or non-violence. It's said to seriously disrupt the person's cycle of birth, death, and rebirth. Some Hindus believe committers of suicide wind up being ghosts walking the earth until the time they would have died naturally, then go to (temporary) hell before reincarnating on earth.[32]

Buddhism doesn't condemn suicide outright but teaches that, like in Hinduism, it also likely will derail one's path to enlightenment, and doing so in anger or other negative mental conditions could make the person worse off in the next life. But there are rare exceptions.[33] In some cases, stronger belief in Buddhism or Taoism may even lead to more suicide. Two China-based scholars, one of whom is affiliated with SUNY Buffalo, launched a study on seventy-four serious suicide attempters who landed in emergency rooms. A third of them believed in reincarnation. Among females, the stronger the belief in reincarnation the stronger the suicide intent. "To some Chinese individuals, being religious is equivalent to being superstitious, and death is a solution to all the problems and the beginning of a new life," write Jie Zhang and Huilan Xu. "Therefore, it is possible that those who got into extremity are likely to think about starting a new life by ending this miserable one quickly." A contributing factor to the depression and suicide is lack of social support. Unlike in Western religions, the authors observe that the majority of Chinese Buddhists and Taoists don't meet regularly as a group.[34] The same is true for Hinduism.[35]

An earlier study compared suicide rates of Singaporean women of Chinese descent, Malay descent, and Indian descent. At 51 suicides per 100,000, Malay women had the lowest rates, and the researchers concluded that was because of their Muslim faith. Ethnic Chinese' and Indians' rate was 112 and 344 per 100,000 respectively. The Indians in Singapore are mostly Hindu.[36] Their high rate indicates the relative laxity in Hindu teaching against such an act. Certain cultural factors among Indians may even encourage it. "People groups of the cultural east and west have vastly different views on the end of life," write Vanderbilt's Andrew Wu and colleagues. Whereas in Western cultures suicide has been associated with shame and cowardice, in the Eastern world it historically has been viewed as an act of nobility and selflessness, "both views of which are linked with the dominant religious and spiritual beliefs of these areas."[37]

Chapter 11

CHURCH LIFTS POOR AND MINORITIES

Whereas Dawn was fifteen she slid into drugs and alcohol, and got pregnant. Three kids and five marriages later, having been beaten, raped, in and out of rehab centers, and in three serious car wrecks, she's doing a lot better. "God kept me," she related. "I am so grateful to God and Jesus, my Lord, for saving me and giving me another chance at a good life with my kids. As of now, I have been involved in church almost two years. My children are thriving in God's house and in His Word. I've noticed my children tend to think of others first. They talk to their friends about what God can do for them. I am so fortunate to have such wonderful children, especially after all they have been through." She's involved in prison ministry, women's ministry, nursing home ministry, the food bank, and her kids' youth group. "We try to be active in everything that concerns spreading God's Word."[1]

Had Dawn the good fortune to find God at a much earlier age, she may have dodged much of that hardship. Church fosters chastity, and chastity fosters domestic stability—instead of domestic violence and economic hardship. About 15 percent of U.S. children under eighteen are classified as living below the poverty line.[2] Much of that poverty results from unmarried teen motherhood, which is tied to widespread sexual activity. That's more likely to occur among the nonreligious or nominally religious. "Studies in our review generally show that those who are religious are less likely to engage in premarital sex or extramarital affairs or to have multiple sexual partners," writes Byron Johnson in Objective Hope.

Of the 38 studies Objective Hope reviewed, 37 showed significant correlations between increased religious involvement and lower likelihood of promiscuous sex, which of course often leads to birth out of wedlock. Only one study showed mixed results, and none found that increased religious participation is linked to promiscuity.[3] Echoing those findings, Rand Corporation researchers conducted a survey confirming that rates of single parenthood are significantly higher for nonreligious persons than religious ones. Those indicating they're "not at all religious" are three times as likely to give birth out of wedlock as those calling themselves "very religious."[4]

Powering the poverty, unmarried teen mothers typically lack good-paying job skills and often cannot work at all because of their childcare responsibilities. They live in cheaper or even substandard housing due to the absence of a spouse's paycheck. Same for those who divorce. Non-churchgoers are more likely to divorce or never marry in the first place. Christine Olson of the Heritage Foundation analyzed data from the National Longitudinal Survey of Youth, comparing the income of churchgoing and non-churchgoing families. Average family income for churchgoers was more than $12,000 higher.[5] And that was based on data from the 1980s and 1990s. With inflation and higher per-capita income, undoubtedly that number is far higher now.

Code of Decency vs. Code of the Street

Elijah Anderson, author of *Code of the Street: Decency, Violence, and the Moral Life of the Inner City*, reports that religious institutions within the inner city try to combat the lure of the street among young Black men, denouncing promiscuity, crime, and drug use. They provide substantial support to church members, fostering among them a "code of decency" that emphasizes family values, civility, and education. UVA's Wilcox and U of U's Wolfinger write that Anderson's research suggests "religious institutions may be one of the key institutional sources of support for relationship-related beliefs and strategies of action that foster marriage in communities where the retreat from marriage is most pronounced."[6]

Urban churches, state Wilcox and Wolfinger, serve as moral and social bulwarks in communities that would see even more social breakdown if not for those places of worship. Strong churches lead to higher rates of marriage which in turn positively impacts health, earnings, and civic engagement of husband and wife. Benefits flow to children who tend to achieve higher levels of education and better social adjustment than children of divorced or never-married parents.[7] Regular public worship improves young Black males' school attendance, job performance, time management, and ability to avoid delinquency.[8]

Married-couple church attendance is higher among Blacks than among Whites or Hispanics, according to Ellison and Wilcox along with Florida State's Amy Burdette.[9] Blacks also engage in at-home religious activities to a greater extent, such as prayer and scripture study. Higher African American religious practice helps offset other socioeconomic factors that negatively impact marriage. Were it not for the strong religiosity of African Americans, marriage rates within that demographic may be lower and out-of-wedlock births higher. In the inner city, parents who attend church at least several times a month are significantly more likely to be married at childbirth, according to Wilcox and Wolfinger. And when unmarried women become pregnant, those who attend church frequently are much more likely to marry the father before giving birth. Among those who don't marry before birth, churchgoing mothers and fathers are significantly more likely to do so within a year of it.[10]

To be sure, divorce rates are higher among Black inner-city residents, even ones who are religious. What explains the "African American religion-marriage paradox" whereby Blacks have higher-than-average church attendance yet higher divorce rates than other racial groups, and lower marriage rates and more out-of-wedlock births? Tremendous socioeconomic factors other than religious attendance impact marriage and out-of-wedlock birth. Recall that religion is by no means the only factor determining well-being. In the inner city are powerful counterweights to the positive influence of religion on marriage, including lower levels of education and income. Also stressing relationships are unemployment, underemployment, and poverty. Another factor is welfare, wherein the state replaces the husband as the primary source of income, discouraging marriage.[11] Welfare reform during the 1990s alleviated this problem, but it still persists.

An additional reason for the paradox: Some churches place less emphasis on marriage than do other churches. Certainly, plenty of them stress the importance of marriage, that sexual relations and childbearing should take place within it, and that sex outside of it is sinful. But this isn't the case everywhere. As touched on two chapters ago, instead of focusing on marriage and family values, certain churches emphasize political themes such as social justice, economic redistribution, and community enfranchisement. They're more tolerant of premarital sex and nonmarital childbearing and may ignore those topics altogether—particularly when many of the congregants are divorced or never married themselves.[12] The social/political focus is what congregants often prefer. "Individuals who are members of a Black church for primarily social or political reasons may pay less attention to the family norms it promotes than individuals who are members for primarily religious or familial reasons," write Wilcox and Wolfinger.[13]

Academic Achievement Among At-Risk Youth

Sixteen-year-old Deion started going to Tree of Life Missionary Baptist Church in Gary, Indiana when he was small. Youth there are surrounded and supported by a community of youths and adults. "At school," he remarked, "you receive encouragement but there is a lot of negativity...At church you know somebody will pick you up if you need it, and there is always a hand on your back, and you always feel it there."[14] Churches are one of the few mainstream institutions ready and willing to reach out and firmly ensconce themselves in crime-ridden and poverty-stricken locales. For boys like Deion, they are places of refuge and beacons of hope in an otherwise bleak world.

In inner cities and other low-income areas of the country, despite multifaceted obstacles such as family disintegration, gang participation, failing schools, joblessness, lack of resources, and prevalence of drugs, many youths manage to rise out of that culture. They stay in school and graduate, avoid drugs and alcohol dependency, stay out of serious trouble, land jobs, marry, and start families. Regnerus and Elder isolated factors behind this. A prominent one is faith-based institutions. "Churches and religious organizations are increasingly being recognized as partners in steering youth away from crime and drug use, and toward educational success," they observe.[15]

In low-income neighborhoods lacking secular institutions that provide social support, religious institutions fill some of that void. It's within them that youth are encouraged to stay out of trouble, work hard, plan for the future, and strive for achievement. Inspiration comes from both their faith and others within the church. They cultivate friendships with like-minded youth.

If high religiosity benefits youth from middle- and upper-income families, then it should benefit low-income students even more, since in many cases they lack the array of extracurricular activities available elsewhere. Sure enough, that's the case according to Regnerus and Elder's study. They used data from Add Health to measure the extent to which students were "on track" in school and whether religious commitment and involvement influenced that.

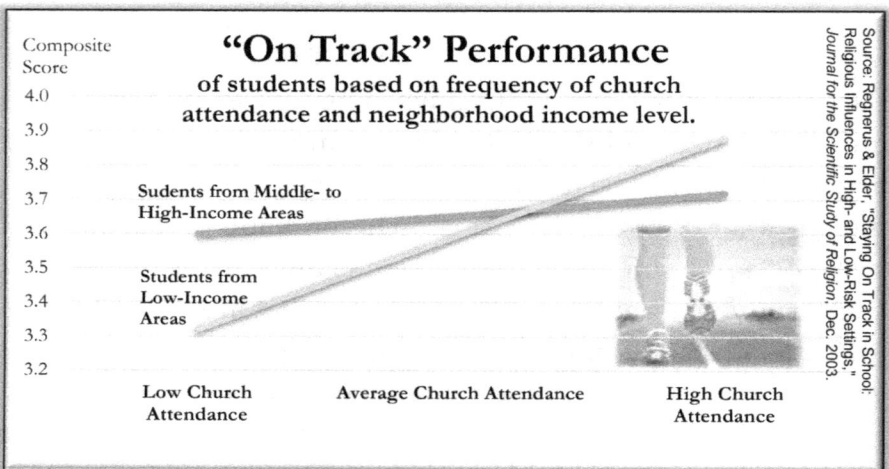

"On Track" Performance
of students based on frequency of church attendance and neighborhood income level.

Composite Score

4.0
3.9
3.8
3.7   Sudents from Middle- to
       High-Income Areas
3.6
3.5
3.4   Students from
       Low-Income
3.3   Areas
3.2

Low Church   Average Church Attendance   High Church
Attendance   Attendance

Source: Regnerus & Elder, "Staying On Track in School: Religious Influences in High- and Low-Risk Settings," *Journal for the Scientific Study of Religion*, Dec. 2003.

Staying on track entails maintaining an adequate GPA, regularly completing homework, avoiding being expelled or suspended, getting along with teachers and classmates, and not skipping class.

The more frequent the churchgoing, the greater the likelihood of staying on track in low- and higher-income communities alike. But in low-income areas, that effect is more pronounced—so much so that as the graph above shows, frequent-churchgoing youth have as good or even better on-track performance than frequent-churchgoing youth in higher-income areas.

In more affluent locales, faith-based institutions compete with a host of other developmental resources for the attention of youth. As mentioned in chapter 8, in low-income communities it's churches that commonly sponsor sports leagues and other neighborhood organizations. Even when they don't, church and belief in God are strong supports in and of themselves. As one inner-city Philadelphia youth put it, referring to herself and her mother, "We support each other. We have a strong relationship with God. God is our support. I don't know—it comes from within. We don't have too many supports. We just don't. They're not there."[16]

Regnerus and Elder add, "Church attendance functions as a protective mechanism in high-risk communities in a way that it does not in low-risk ones, stimulating educational resilience in the lives of at-risk youth. We argue that adolescents' participation in religious communities—which often constitute the key sources of neighborhood developmental resources—reinforces messages about working hard and staying out of trouble, orients them toward a positive future, and builds a transferable skill set of commitments and routines."

What is it about active worship that so positively influences academic progress?" Regnerus and Elder cite positive role models that youth are exposed to at places of worship, in addition to various support networks. The mere process of attending worship services has a lot to do with it. As mentioned in chapter 8, simply having to get up on Sunday mornings and go to church, and learn to sit still there, can have beneficial effects elsewhere. Church attendance requires commitment, diligence, and routine—qualities that apply to the academic world. "The ritual practice of rising and going to church or mass, and so forth—whether compelled by one's own faith or one's parents' demands—commits a youth to a practice and routine, a skill that translates into tools needed for academic success," write Regnerus and Elder. This may partly explain why private religiosity, in which the person considers him- or herself religious but doesn't regularly attend church, is less associated with better academic performance.[17]

Toldson and Anderson provide further confirmation that it's not enough just to believe. Ivory Toldson is editor-in-chief of *The Journal of Negro Education*, professor at Howard University, and senior research analyst for the Congressional Black Caucus Foundation. He and Howard professor and associate dean Kenneth Alonzo Anderson found that students' participation in religious activities has a much stronger effect on academic success than merely how important they consider religion in their lives. Black students' ratings of the importance of religion (as opposed to churchgoing) weren't even associated with academic success. The investigators crunched numbers from a national survey of 6,795 eighth and tenth graders titled "Monitoring the Future: A Continuing Study of American Youth." They write, "Clearly, results revealed that Black students who had a positive self-concept, positive feelings about school, parents involved with their education, fewer disciplinary referrals, and higher grades were more likely to participate in religious services more frequently." They recommend that Black churches do even more to promote education, which may take the form of routinely monitoring students' grades, providing incentives to do well in school, and interceding on behalf of youth suspended from school.[18]

The authors note that their results don't necessarily confirm that greater religiosity leads to higher grades. They suggest academically successful students may be more religiously inclined, or some external factor could be influencing both religion and grades, such as actions of parents.

Combatting Crime and Delinquency

John Pridmore was born in London's East End. Growing up without faith and in a broken home, as a teen he slid into a life of delinquency. In and out of prison, and mesmerized by the lure of riches, sex, and power, he became a full-fledged gangster with the top organized crime figures in London. "I slowly obtained everything the world says makes you happy. I had the penthouse apartment, the sports cars, more money than I could spend. But inside, there was this overwhelming sense of emptiness." Once at a nightclub, with brass knuckles he hit someone and thought he killed him. "As I drove home that night, I thought, what have I become, that I could kill someone and not even care?" When he got home he felt God speaking to his heart, but apparently, not in an upbeat way. "I knew I was going to hell." He cried out for another chance. In the first prayer of his life he uttered, "Up to now, all I've done is take from you, God. Now I want to give." His disposition changed then and there. "That emptiness, which always filled my heart, was suddenly filled with the love of God, the Holy Spirit. And in that moment I knew God could love someone like me." Not long after, he went on a religious retreat where he had another spiritual awakening, and went to confession. "That part of me that could never be redeemed, was suddenly redeemed."[19]

Pridmore went on to become an internationally known speaker and author. As his story attests, prayer, faith, and church are powerful crime-stoppers. They're instrumental in turning around the lives of criminals and thwarting would-be felons from ever going down that path in the first place.

Studies bear this out. When Richard Freeman of Harvard and Harry Holzer of Michigan State analyzed the results of a survey consisting of more than 2,300 interviews of males age 16-24 residing in low-income areas of Boston, Philadelphia, and Chicago, they noticed a prominent pattern: churchgoing was helping to keep them out of crime. They questioned whether it was church making them that way or whether simply "good kids" tend to go to church.

They concluded that yes, churchgoing plays an independent role in keeping young people upright amid the crime-ridden streets.[20] Another study compared men from an inner-city community who eventually landed in prison and those who didn't. The contrast was stark: the prison-avoiders for the most part were regular church-goers, whereas the majority of prisoners either had never attended church or stopped going around the age of ten.[21]

Evidence is abundant that religiosity among at-risk populations helps stave off delinquency and deviant behavior. This is the case even without strong social pressure in the surrounding community against such behavior. Of 46 studies on crime and delinquency sur-veyed in Objective Hope, 37 indicate religious activity is associated with less misconduct. Only one had the opposite conclusion, one found mixed results, and seven found no association.[22]

Churchgoing youth have a 39 percent lower likelihood of com-mitting a non-drug crime than non-churchgoers. For drug-related crime it's a 46 percent lower likelihood, and for drug dealing 57 percent lower. And in accord with the pattern found throughout this book, mere religious belief isn't enough. It's churchgoing that's key. "Attitudinal measures of religious devotion (one's response to how important of a role religion plays in his or her life) is not sig-nificantly linked to reductions in juvenile delinquency," write Byron Johnson of Baylor and Marc Siegel of UPenn.[23]

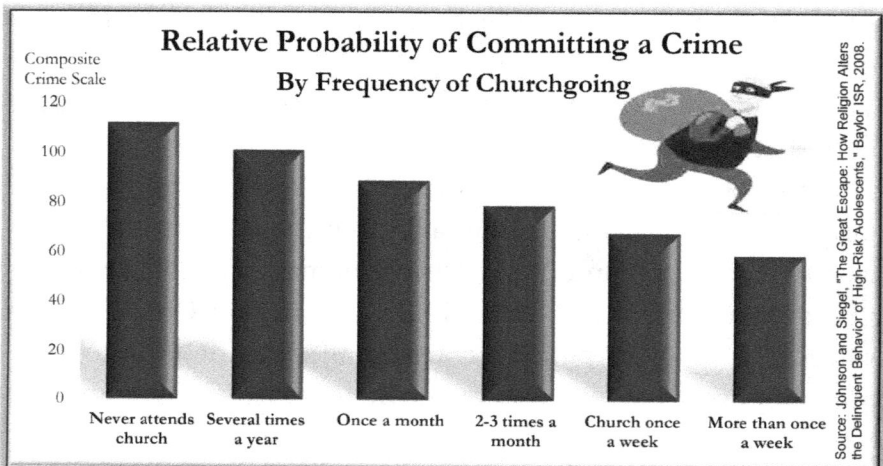

Relative Probability of Committing a Crime
By Frequency of Churchgoing

Composite Crime Scale

Never attends church · Several times a year · Once a month · 2-3 times a month · Church once a week · More than once a week

Source: Johnson and Siegel, "The Great Escape: How Religion Alters the Delinquent Behavior of High-Risk Adolescents," Baylor ISR, 2008.

The more religious the parents, the less their kids fall into delinquency, according to the National Study of Youth and Religion.[24] The kids also have more involvement in other community activities and fewer delinquent-prone friends. And delinquent youth who embrace church not only often amend their ways but gravitate toward a productive career.[25]

On the home front, more churchgoing means more peace. Men attending church at least once a week are as much as 60 percent less likely than non-churchgoers to physically abuse their partner, report Ellison along with Kristin Anderson of Western Washington University. (That's based on self-reports of violence. Using partner reports, the figure is 49 percent.) Women attending once a week or more are 44 percent less likely to behave violently toward their partners (35 percent for partner-reported). Even women attending once a month are less prone to violence. Reasons the researchers offer for church's protective effect on domestic violence include positive messages of intimate bonds and family relations, informal contacts with other church members, and outright condemnation of family violence at some churches.[26]

Faith-Based Rehab Programs

Once felons finish their prison sentence they can have a hard time readjusting, often sliding back into crime. Many programs throughout the United States aim to prevent that eventuality. Objective Hope reports that faith-based ones stand out. An example is Kairos Horizons (now called Kairos Prison Ministry International) which seeks to improve behavior and boost literacy. Compared with the control group, those in the program generally were convicted of more severe crimes and had longer sentences. Even so, Kairos participants as a whole had fewer disciplinary problems and attained higher literacy.

Prison Fellowship Ministries assists prisoners and former prisoners through an extensive network of church-based volunteers. One study featured in Objective Hope evaluated former convicts who participated in a two-week seminar conducted by PFM, designed to support their faith and enhance leadership skills as volunteer prison ministers. Compared with a matched control group, during the eight- to fourteen-year follow-up period, the seminar participants had significantly lower rates of recidivism. In Brazil, inmates at the Braganca prison got vocational training and skills-building to help better prepare them for release. At the Humaita prison the emphasis was religious programs in an effort to "kill the criminal and save the person." After three years the Humaita recidivism rate was significantly lower than that of Braganca.[27]

Chapter 12

NOT ALL SPIRITUALITY IS EQUAL

Eighteen-year-old Mia grew up in a Christian family but never prayed nor had an active relationship with God. Beset since she was eight with anxiety, obsessive-compulsive disorder, depression, and panic attacks, she hardly left her house. "I just was like trapped inside myself; trapped inside a bubble and I just wanted to be set free. There was a point where I told my parents that I'm done. Like is my life gonna be like this forever? I can't live my life like this. I had to go to a therapist three times a week. I got put on medication." She developed an eating disorder and anorexia. "I was nasty and rude to my family. I pushed them away. I got in fights and arguments with them every day…I never thought about God or Jesus or anything other than myself…I didn't care about my health. I just wanted to be skinny…Anorexia isn't just a health problem, it's a mental illness. And it consumed me."

One time she was listening to a podcast on New Age practices such as mindfulness meditation, "law of attraction" manifestation techniques, and chakra cleansing. They "don't depend on God at all. It's all dependent on you, it's all about you. And I got caught in that. I was trying to meditate to chakra cleanse, to try to be more balanced, and I was trying to control my destiny." Some time later she came across a video warning Christians against dabbling in the New Age—and she still considered herself a Christian. She watched more such videos and realized she was being pulled away from God, depending on herself to fix things and not depending on Him. "At this time my brother was reading the Bible and I was like, 'Oh that's cool, I want to try to start reading the Bible because I wanted to get closer to God and Jesus.'" She started at the beginning of the Bible with the book of Genesis but it felt like a chore. She then came across Internet videos of teachings and preachers of the Gospel, which inspired her to start perusing it. "Reading the Gospel completely changed my view of the world...and how I treat people...For so long I was so focused on myself and what people think of me. But I now know that none of that matters. The only thing that matters is what God thinks of you...I used to be so afraid of death and like, 'What if I die? What if this happens?' And I'm not afraid of it anymore. I'm looking forward to that day where I can meet Jesus and I can live with him and spend eternity by his side in the kingdom of heaven."[1]

Mia is a prime example of what so often happens to lukewarm Christians. They're susceptible to mental disorders. For a way out, instead of returning to their childhood faith, they go New Age. They're "spiritual but not religious" (SBNR), rejecting organized religion but believing in some sort of higher power.

The higher power can encompass a range of things including the deistic concept of a creator of the universe who no longer is actively involved in its affairs, to the theistic God who's actively involved, to Jesus minus his Church, to Buddha, to Hindu gods, to an impersonal life-force that's said to connect all things. An SBNR may often pray privately, or may not. While some definitions of SBNR include nearly any kind of meaningful activity without even implying anything supernatural, our definition here does imply belief in the supernatural. Also called self-transcendence, SBNR additionally may entail efforts to connect with the other-worldly, such as prayer or meditation, but doesn't include churchgoing and/ or other forms of conventional religious practices.

Are there wellness benefits of SBNR? Certainly, at-home prayer and/or meditation—even secular meditation—can reduce stress and anxiety.[2] Nevertheless, few studies have been conducted on the long-term wellness benefits of SBNR because of difficulty in defining the concept. "Spirituality means so many things to so many people that to do really good research, you need to clarify what is meant by that," said Tyler VanderWeele. One thing is certain: being spiritual *and* religious is better for health. He emphasizes that it's the communal aspects of worship that are key.[3] That's confirmed in a study he carried out with Ying Chen and Eric Kim at Harvard. *Crossroads* calls it an "extraordinary rigorous analysis" that provides "strong evidence for the health benefits of gathering together for community worship and prayer." Those benefits include less depression, anxiety, hopelessness, loneliness, and alcoholism, as well as greater life satisfaction, purpose in life, and physical health.[4]

UT Austin's Marc Musick along with two UM-Ann Arbor colleagues in the *Journal of Health and Social Behavior* affirm the communal benefits of being both spiritual and religious, indicating that simply praying and reading scripture but avoiding regularly attending worship services appears to have little or no benefit for longevity. Activities associated with church such as communal prayer, singing hymns, receiving communion, lectoring, ushering, greeting, and choir singing involve active participation and social interaction—something not possible when only staying home.[5]

A study led by Marilyn Baetz of the University of Saskatchewan confirms high spiritual values without churchgoing is associated with higher rates of mood and anxiety disorders. This doesn't necessarily mean the spiritual values cause them. Baetz and her colleagues suggest psychiatric disorders could prompt a formerly non-spiritual person to search for meaning, strength, and understanding of life's difficulties through spirituality, which helps explains why SBNRs have higher rates of mental disorders. Mia was a perfect example. "Religion or spirituality may not be as highly valued during a current psychiatric illness, but over time, these values may help individuals grow through their experiences," write the scholars.[6] A separate study done in the United Kingdom disclosed SBNRs generally have worse mental health not only compared with churchgoers but also compared with the neither spiritual nor religious. As a possible explanation, "they are caught up in an existential search that is driven by their emotional distress."[7] This goes hand-in-hand with what's discussed in this book's introduction: many people ignore God during good times and only seek Him during bad times—which is one reason why God allows pain and suffering in the world. (Note that the U.K. study also concluded that, contrary to findings in the U.S., secular persons didn't have greater mental disorders than religious persons in the U.K. with the exception of drug and alcohol dependency. The study authors say it may be because religiosity is significantly lower in the U.K., resulting in an absence of social support for religious persons.)

UW-Madison's Chaeyoon Lim and Harvard's Robert Putnam state that private religious practices such as at-home prayer and spiritual reading aren't significantly related to life satisfaction. "Combined with the findings on congregational friendship and private religious practices, this suggests that religious belonging, rather than religious meaning, is central to the religion-life satisfaction nexus."[8] A possible exception is with adolescents. Chen and VanderWeele found that non-churchgoing teens who pray or meditate daily have better emotional processing and fewer health problems than churchgoing teens. Ironically this may reflect the latter attending church out of obedience to parents rather than out of personal conviction, whereas the teens who pray daily at home do it because they really want to. Nevertheless, the churchgoing teens scored higher on life satisfaction, positive affectivity, non-smoking, and chastity.[9]

Also among teens, SBNR boosts the risks of running afoul of both parents and the law. In his study "Secrets and Lies: Adolescent Religiosity and Concealing Information from Parents," Scott Desmond of IUPUC looked at the relationship between religiosity and morality among adolescents. Those who publicly worship and place high importance on religion are more likely to say it's less acceptable to break moral rules, such as substance abuse and delinquency. But adolescents who identify as SBNR are more accepting of breaking those rules.[10]

The Spiritual But Not Religious are Missing Out

SBNRs lack the social component of traditional religion, which appears to be a huge factor in enhancing wellness. It's baked into the human condition. In previous times, people lived in close-knit communities where they knew many local people well and interacted with them often. The renowned French sociologist Émile Durkheim wrote of the importance of this in maintaining well-being.[11] This arrangement still is the case in many small towns and in developing countries. A typical household in a lower-income country often has a steady stream of visitors stopping by unannounced to chat, be they neighbors, friends, or relatives. However, in modern suburban and urban society where anonymity is common and people are more transient, close-knit community is much rarer. This relative lack of personal interaction is one reason why depression and other mental disorders are generally higher in high-income countries.

People strive to re-create close-knit communities through clubs, service organizations, sports groups, and other activities. But often they fall short. What can re-create them in a more meaningful way are churches, thanks in part to core values congregants share—as Clay's story in chapter 2 about finding his church community attests. Musick and colleagues write, "Members of religious institutions share a common set of beliefs, meet regularly, share a common commitment to help other members if needed, provide and enforce a framework for acceptable behavior, and work to maintain the overall functioning of the group through volunteer activities and contributions."[12] The significance of a church community is larger than the individuals who comprise it.

If you're SBNR and move to a new town or city, you may be at a loss in making friends or even interacting with others on a regular basis. In rejecting organized religion you're encumbering your ability to join a close-knit community. Absent are the new friends, camaraderie, and social activities you could have enjoyed—and the health benefits. The same holds true for the neither spiritual nor religious. You may chime in, "What if I don't believe anything they believe? I don't want to show up somewhere and pretend to believe in something just to be part of a group. That would be phony." See the last chapter for compelling reasons to believe.

Organized worship also makes sense because otherwise, chances are it would be disorganized worship. Assume you're SBNR and follow Jesus Christ. Are you self-disciplined enough to regularly read the Bible and pray to him, especially Sunday mornings? If not, you need the structure of organized worship. If you do have that self-discipline, you'll likely eventually feel compelled to worship him with others and get the support of a faith community. In the Bible Jesus was clear in his intention to establish a church ("…and on this rock I will build my church," Matthew 16:18), which in the original Greek—*ecclesia*—means a regularly convoked assembly or gathering. It's like little candles coming together to form a big fire.[13] The Old Testament establishes that God absolutely wishes to be formally worshiped, with His detailed commands to construct altars, build the Holy Temple, give obeisance, offer sacrifice, and carry out other rituals. In the New Testament Jesus the Son sacrifices himself to the Father, and orders that we consume his body and blood under the forms of consecrated bread and wine. That only can be done in formal worship. So in addition to the fellowship you get in such a setting, which has been proven to be good for your wellness, you get God's graces. That's got to be good for your wellness, too.

It's not just the benefits of communal worship that SBNRs are forfeiting. They're exempting themselves from the responsibilities, obligations, and associated self-discipline of organized religion. Those responsibilities may seem annoying or even difficult, but that's what delayed gratification is all about. "Right now, spiritual means basically anything you want it to mean," said Koenig. "And it usually means doing whatever you want to do, and ignoring the religious laws and doctrines that tell you what not to do. They basically want the benefits without any of the costs."[14] It's a recipe for trouble down the road.

While SBNRs tend to score higher on receptiveness to new ideas and experiences, they score lower on self-control and conscientiousness. That's the conclusion of the University of Miami's McCullough and Willoughby who analyzed data from the Self-Transcendence scale of the Temperament and Character Inventory, a survey that measures spirituality as opposed to traditional religious beliefs and practices. They observe that certain aspects of religious beliefs, behaviors, rituals, and institutions engender self-control. This could stem from sets of rules inspired by an omniscient deity, from the perception one's actions are monitored by that deity, and/or from the self-discipline needed to regularly attend formal religious worship.[15]

Intrinsically Good

Formal religious worship is key. But even then, if your heart isn't into it, you won't get as much out of it. Studies show that church-goers of weak faith don't experience the mental and physical health benefits on the scale churchgoers of strong faith enjoy. So don't treat church as a social club. Don't have the attitude that you're there to lower your blood pressure. Instead, do it for reasons such as these:

- to worship God on the Sabbath day.
- to offer God prayers of praise, thanksgiving, contrition, petition, and intercession.
- to learn more about God and his teachings.
- to deepen your faith and advance your spiritual development.
- to seek God's guidance when making decisions.
- to strive to experience the presence of the Divine.
- to acknowledge your sins.
- to seek inner peace.
- to work toward the goal of happiness in the next life.

Persons who have the above in mind are what scholars call "intrinsically religious"—attending church based on a desire for spiritual transformation and a stronger and more meaningful relationship with God. To be sure, being intrinsically religious isn't necessarily an all-or-nothing phenomenon. There are varying degrees of intrinsic religiosity, depending on where one is on one's faith journey.

On the other hand there are the "extrinsically religious" or those who attend for reasons external to what church is supposed to be about, and who aren't so committed to their faith in the way the intrinsically religious are. People frequent the pews for all kinds of reasons that don't have much to do with actual worship of God. For the extrinsically religious, the main motivation for church involves factors such as these:

- a family tradition.
- a cultural tradition.
- for inclusion in an established religion, denomination, or culture.
- to socialize and attend social activities.
- to participate in a church-sponsored laity group.
- to make friends and/or spend time with friends.
- to network—increase contacts for job or business opportunities.
- out of a feeling of obligation to parents, spouse, or other family members.
- to maintain a routine carried out since childhood.
- to engage in community outreach and volunteer/charitable activities.
- to project an outward image of being a churchgoer in communities where active worship is a social norm.
- to please one's spouse.
- to seek a romantic partner or spouse.
- out of a preference to get married in a church setting.
- to foster religiosity in one's children—where the parent views religion as a good thing and a moral foundation for children even though the parent may not be particularly religious.
- to enjoy church music, art, architecture, rituals, ceremony, and the like.
- as an avenue to sing or play an instrument.
- to listen to dynamic speakers/preachers.
- and last but not least, out of a sole desire to improve your mental and/or physical health.

Mind you, those are all still very good reasons to go to church. If they're what motivate you, then by all means go for it. Everyone is at a different point on their spiritual journey. Perhaps you're just starting out, and you want to believe but can't bring yourself to do so yet. The key is to educate yourself on the tremendous evidence of God's existence, on His love and mercy, and on how He wants to be worshipped—all the while attending church each week with the expectation that sooner or later, the Holy Spirit will build that faith in you. Or, perhaps you started your journey long ago but don't feel you're advancing. Chances are you're not giving it the attention it needs; maybe you're just going through the motions each Sunday but doing little or no praying or spiritual reading during the rest of the week. Now's the time to start. For help with that, see the last chapter.

Naturally, intrinsically religious persons attend church for many of the above reasons, but those are secondary to the first set of reasons. They don't do it for the mental and physical health benefits. But they're rewarded with those nevertheless—more so than extrinsically religious persons. Studies have found that compared with extrinsics, intrinsics generally have lower levels of depression, anxiety, stress, and guilt. This was noticed as far back as the 1960s when Harvard psychologists Gordon Allport and J. Michael Ross carried out a study juxtaposing intrinsic and extrinsic religious attitudes. Wrote Allport, "I feel equally sure that mental health is facilitated by an intrinsic, but not an extrinsic, religious orientation."[16]

Intrinsic religiosity speeds recovery from illness. Koenig and colleagues studied physically ill, hospitalized older patients. Though they were there for physical treatment, depression rates among them were higher than among community-dwelling older adults, and depression tends to delay recovery of physical illness. The investigators measured patients' level of religiosity. The intrinsics recovered faster than extrinsics. Simple church attendance and private religious activities alone didn't affect recovery times; only when coupled with intrinsic religiosity was there an impact.[17] In the study mentioned in chapter 2 of open-heart surgery patients at Dartmouth-Hitchcock Medical Center, the death rate six months later was 11 percent among those who were "not at all," "slightly," or "fairly" religious. Among the "deeply" religious the death rate was zero.[18]

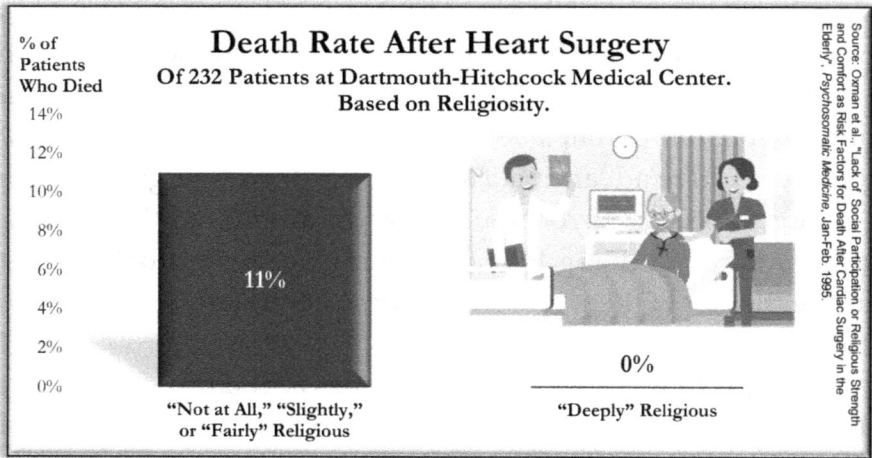

Death Rate After Heart Surgery
Of 232 Patients at Dartmouth-Hitchcock Medical Center.
Based on Religiosity.

% of Patients Who Died

14%
12%
10%
8%
6%
4%
2%
0%

11%

0%

"Not at All," "Slightly," or "Fairly" Religious

"Deeply" Religious

Source: Oman et al., "Lack of Social Participation or Religious Strength and Comfort as Risk Factors for Death After Cardiac Surgery in the Elderly", *Psychosomatic Medicine*, Jan-Feb. 1995.

Writing in the 1990s and early 2000s, Patrick Fagan cites academic studies concluding that intrinsic religiosity is associated with moral standards, discipline, conscientiousness, consistency, and responsibility. Surprisingly, extrinsic motivation "is often linked to self-indulgence, indolence, and a lack of dependability." Rubbing salt into the wounds, he observes that according to studies, extrinsics are more likely to be self-centered as well as "dogmatic, authoritarian, and less responsible."[19] Ouch. Could those words be true? Many of those studies are from the 1960s, 1970s, and early 1980s. Back then, far more Americans went to church than today. It was more of a nationwide cultural norm. Even blockheads and racists darkened church doors. It was when churchgoers generally were less educated than non-churchgoers; now that situation is reversed as pointed out in chapter 8. Allport's 1967 study sought to discover whether the level of racial prejudice differed between the extrinsically and intrinsically religious. He determined that intrinsics were the least racially prejudiced. Among infrequent churchgoers and extrinsically motivated churchgoers, racial prejudice was highest.[20] Thankfully, racism is far less prevalent today than in the 1960s and where it does exist, we can make an educated guess that those persons generally go to church only occasionally or not at all.

These days most extrinsics are nice, upstanding people. Even if folks are mainly in church for health and wellness benefits, that's a great incentive to get them through the door and involved in various church-sponsored activities. Then, if they do their homework and are open to the Holy Spirit, hopefully they'll transition to intrinsic.

Intrinsics generally have less anxiety over the ups and downs of life—and death. Extrinsics tend to be more worried about death not only compared with intrinsics but also compared with the nonreligious. Among college students (who are so commonly studied thanks to academics' proximity to them) intrinsics on average have higher discipline and self-control, dependability, and GPAs.[21] And as reported by Panagiota Darvyri and colleagues at the University of Athens, intrinsics tend to:

- have better overall physical and mental health.
- under stress, have lower blood pressure.
- have lower rates of anxiety and depression.
- be more conscientious.
- have significantly higher spiritual well-being, which is associated with hope.
- have positive moods.

Being extrinsically religious can be associated with love of worldly things—attending church not out of a desire to focus on the spiritual but out of a desire to enhance one's personal, social, business, or other temporal aspect of one's life. "Religion directed toward some end other than God, or the transcendent, typically degenerates into a rationalization for the pursuit of other ends such as status, personal security, self-justification, or sociability," admonishes Fagan.[22] As stated in 1 John 2:15-16,

> "Do not love the world or the things in the world. If anyone loves the world, the love of the Father is not in him. For all that is in the world—the desires of the flesh and the desires of the eyes and pride in possessions—is not from the Father but is from the world."

Or Colossians 3:2,

> "Set your minds on things that are above, not on
> things that are on earth."

Strong words indeed. They evoke the perils of fixating on Levels 1 and 2 happiness. That said, it's still greatly preferable to be extrinsically religious and attend church than not attend at all—especially if you're doing it for such reasons as fostering faith in your children, making friends, enjoying music and art, volunteering to help the poor, and/or finding a romantic partner; it's far better to seek a soulmate at the church scene than the bar scene.

Chapter 13

SUPERNATURAL GRACES

Kathy was a human resources manager at a nonprofit. One day upon undergoing a routine mammogram, the X-ray showed a lump. She got scared and upset. Surgeons recommended a biopsy. Kathy turned to prayer. At the office, two co-workers began praying for her, following the ancient Christian practice of laying hands on her. "They just prayed and prayed and prayed, and I was praying to myself. It was powerful!," declared Kathy. On the day of the biopsy, unbeknownst to her, church friends fervently prayed for a miracle. A church elder arrived and prayed along with her. "I was hoping the lump would be gone, but I had also accepted the fact that, whatever God decided, it was His plan," remembered Kathy. Doctors ran a mammogram that morning but this time found no lump. Then came two more X-ray sessions by two different radiologists. Comparing that day's X-rays with the original ones, they were baffled. They went ahead with the biopsy. And still, the lump was nowhere to be found. "Do you believe in the power of prayer?," asked the technician. "Do I ever!," Kathy exclaimed.[1]

The above was recounted by physician and Georgetown University School of Medicine professor Dale Matthews. He's unusual in that not many professionals who study religion and health are so vocal about the idea that churchgoers could be receiving direct or indirect help from the supernatural realm. Matthews even wrote a book on it: *The Faith Factor: Proof of the Healing Power of Prayer*.

In identifying what it is about churchgoing that's so beneficial for mental and physical health, the academic literature points to social interaction associated with church, the sense of meaning and purpose, the giving of time and money to charitable causes, and other naturalistic explanations. Academicians focus on science, not on the supernatural. But any believer knows that supernaturalistic explanations abound. There are countless documented medical miracles doctors can't figure out. Back in 1993 scholars assembled a database of 1,385 medical journal articles documenting what medical professionals call spontaneous remissions; the number must be far higher now. Many of them are under the category of "miraculous healings" such as those that occur from bathing in the waters of Lourdes, France where the Blessed Virgin Mary is said to have appeared in 1858.[2] If there's extraordinary supernatural help like this, then it's reasonable to presume ordinary supernatural help over the course of one's churchgoing life. More common are the subtle ways God helps those who pray, be it through an improved family situation, state of mind, prayer life, living condition, or health status. If you praise and worship Him, He's bound to return the favor.

When you're sick or disabled, prayers asking for healing won't necessarily have the outcome you hope for. God's main concern is your spiritual health so you can be with Him in heaven someday. For God, your state in the next world which is eternal is much more important than your bodily health and happiness in this world which are ephemeral. If God thinks better health will facilitate a greater devotion to Him, such as being able to attend church more regularly or volunteer to help the poor more often, then He may grant you that gift. But if it instead prompts you to indulge in fun, entertainment, fast cars, sleek smartphones, and other things that distract you from Him and likely lead you into sin, then He may not grant you any special favors in the area of health. He may even allow you to suffer to some extent, perhaps as a wake-up call.

People often seek out God during hard times while ignoring Him during good times. Suffering can bring someone closer to God through such things as building character, searching for a greater good, finding meaning and purpose, seeking comfort in prayer, and evoking sympathy for others. Jesus says in the Gospels, "If anyone wishes to come after me, he must deny himself and take up his cross daily and follow me." (Luke 9:23) Taking up the cross means suffering for Him.

So will prayers bring physical healing? Sometimes yes, sometimes no. Nevertheless, separate from the thousands of conventional studies on the religion-health relationship, far fewer in number are studies testing the effectiveness of prayers in recovering from ailments. In these randomized trials of prayer, as they're called, researchers designate persons to pray for the recovery of certain hospitalized patients. It's known as intercessory prayer, where those praying intercede for the patients. The latter typically don't know they're being prayed for. Parallel to them is a control group of patients for whom there are no designated intercessors. Of course, family and friends not part of the study may be praying for control-group patients but there's no way the researchers can influence that.

Such studies are wrought with uncertainties because in addition to the inability to eliminate prayers for the control group, no one knows the detailed workings of God or the supernatural world. With hierarchies of multitudes of angels, fallen angels, saints, souls, and realms, the supernatural world must be inordinately multifaceted and complex—far more so than our world. How could we possibly subject it to academic scrutiny when we know so little about it—and when we know so little about God apart from what's revealed in the Bible and in nature? As stated in Isaiah 55:8, "For my thoughts are not your thoughts, neither are your ways my ways, declares the Lord." God works in mysterious ways. But does He respond to contrived prayer, which is essentially what these studies are? No one knows.

Moreover the studies involve intercessors from various religions in addition to New Age-type spirituality including energy healing. This raises questions as to whether all religions are equal in the sight of God. Each has its own idea of the nature of God and of how God wants us to worship Him and live our lives. They all contradict one another and two contradictory ideas logically cannot each be true. For example if one religion champions reincarnation while another teaches that each person only has one life on earth, both can't be right. Hindus believe there are many gods. At least one religion—Theravada Buddhism—holds there's no personal God or gods. Does God act upon a Buddhist's prayers in the same way He acts upon the prayers of a Christian, who affirms the existence and exaltation of Him? And among Christian intercessors, does God respond to a lukewarm Christian in the same way He responds to a fervent believer?

Whatever the case, the majority of randomized trials of prayer actually show a positive health effect. Santa Clara University's John Astin and colleagues examined twenty-three studies on the effect of prayer on physical healing, reporting their results in the *Annals of Internal Medicine*. Thirteen found a positive effect, nine no effect, and one a negative effect.[3] Another study of studies led by Leanne Roberts at Oxford found positive effects of prayer for those at high risk of death—i.e. postponing death—but didn't see differences between prayer groups and control groups regarding the clinical state of patients, or medical complications. The researchers write, "The evidence presented so far is interesting enough to justify further study into the human aspects of the effects of prayer. However it is impossible to prove or disprove in trials any supposed benefit that derives from God's response to prayer."[4]

Psychiatrist Daniel Benor, author of *Spiritual Healing: Scientific Validation of a Healing Revolution*, performed a comprehensive review of many dozens of studies and narrowed them down to the well-designed ones. Of those, about three-quarters found a healing effect of prayer.[5] Now *that's* impressive.

Prayer Works

Cardiologist Randolph Byrd of UC San Francisco in the 1980s carried out one of the first prominent studies of intercessory prayer. It involved 393 patients in a coronary care unit at San Francisco General Hospital, about half of whom were prayed for by designated persons. A mix of Protestants and Catholics, the intercessors prayed daily for certain patients' rapid recovery and prevention of complications. Neither the patients nor medical personnel knew who were being prayed for. The control group members weren't prayed for by anyone involved in the study. Over the course of ten months Byrd monitored each patient, grading his or her condition as good, intermediate, or bad. Of the 192 in the prayed-for group and 201 in the control group, following are the health results:

	Prayed-for group:	Control group:
Good:	163	147
Mixed:	2	10
Bad:	27	44

Eighty-five percent of the prayer group patients were designated as "good" versus only 73 percent in the control group. And the prayer group had only 14 percent "bad" designations versus 22 percent in the control. Byrd observed, "The prayer group had less congestive heart failure, required less diuretic and antibiotic therapy, had fewer episodes of pneumonia, had fewer cardiac arrests, and were less frequently intubated and ventilated."[6] Ellison and Levin write, "For findings such as these, neither the behavioral and psychosocial constructs discussed above nor the possibility of a salutary placebo effect seem to offer feasible explanations."[7] Perhaps it was divine intervention after all.

Naturally there was a lot of skepticism about Byrd's groundbreaking study. So about ten years later a team of researchers sought to replicate it. Like Byrd's, their test subjects were coronary care patients, this time 1,013 of them. The location was the Mid America Heart Institute at Saint Luke's Hospital in Kansas City. The Protestant and Catholic intercessors were given first names of patients as they got admitted to the hospital, and prayed daily for each for twenty-eight days. To determine health outcomes the team used a scoring system that rated conditions ranging from excellent to catastrophic; for example 1 point was assigned for heart catheterization, 4 points for coronary bypass surgery, 5 for heart attack, and

6 for death. The points were added up, so the lower the score the healthier the patient. Results: the prayer group's mean score was 6.24. For the control group it was 6.97. The prayed-for patients were healthier. The authors concluded, "Remote, intercessory prayer was associated with lower CCU (coronary care unit) course scores. This result suggests that prayer may be an effective adjunct to standard medical care."

Another study sought to measure the effects of intercessory prayer and of "distant positive visualization." The latter is a power-of-positive-thinking technique in which someone generates mental images in an effort to bring about physical or psychological healing in someone else. The test subjects were hemodialysis patients with end-stage renal disease. While researchers didn't find a significant effect of intercessory prayer or positive visualization, patients who expected to receive intercessory prayer reported feeling significantly better than patients who expected to receive positive visualization.[8]

Creative Cases of Prayer

Prayer investigators have gotten innovative: a study tested the effects of intercessory prayer on animals. As described in "The Effect of Intercessory Prayer on Wound Healing in Nonhuman Primates," twenty-two bush babies (a.k.a. galagos, which are small nocturnal primates native to Africa) exhibited chronic self-injurious behavior with resulting wounds. All were treated with L-tryptophan which helps build proteins, but one group had daily intercessory prayer for four weeks and the other did not. Results: the prayed-for animals underwent a reduction in wound size compared with the control group. The prayer group also enjoyed improvements in other metrics including a greater increase in red blood cells and hemoglobin. The lesson: don't neglect to pray for your pets.[9]

Another unusual prayer study consisted of one-person, retroactive prayer for patients with bloodstream infections. It was published in the prestigious *BMJ* (British Medical Journal), attesting that the medical establishment takes these studies seriously.

Instead of many people praying, just one offsite person prayed for the well-being and full recovery of the intervention group. Retro-active prayer entails praying for a good outcome of something that happened in the past, without the intercessor previously knowing the result. For example, a high school student takes a biology test in the morning and immediately gets back the results. Her mother, accustomed to praying for her to do well on tests, this time forgets to pray beforehand. No matter—she prays in the afternoon (not yet knowing the test result) that her daughter scored well that morning. A person can do that with God, who's outside time and space. For Him, time isn't linear.

> "With the Lord a day is like a thousand years, and
> a thousand years are like a day." (2 Peter 3:8)

Retroactive prayer is even consistent with quantum mechanics; based on the "delayed choice quantum eraser" experiment, an observer of subatomic particles apparently can influence how those particles behaved in the past. As Albert Einstein wrote, "For people like us who believe in physics, the separation between past, present and future has only the importance of an admittedly tenacious illusion."[10]

Leonard Leibovici of the Rabin Medical Center in Israel conducted the study. It involved 3,393 patients, randomizing them into an intervention group and control group. None of them knew about the study, and certainly not during the time of their ailment—which would have been impossible because the praying didn't take place until much later. Their bloodstream infections were diagnosed from 1990 to 1996. However, the prayer intervention didn't take place until 2000. The single intercessor, who had no idea of the patients' health outcomes, was given a list of first names of those in the intervention group. The intercessor said a short prayer for the group as a whole, petitioning for a swift recovery. So the intervention was performed four to ten years after the infections. Leibovici, who also didn't previously know the patients' outcomes, after the prayer researched their mortality rates, length of hospital stays, and duration of fevers.

The result? The prayer seemed to work. For the intervention group, mortality was 28.1 percent (475 patients died out of 1,691). For the control group it was 30.2 percent (514 out of 1,702 died). The hospital stays and duration of fevers were "significantly shorter" in the intervention group. Leibovici writes, "Remote, retroactive intercessory prayer can improve outcomes in patients with a blood-stream infection. This intervention is cost effective, probably has no adverse effects, and should be considered for clinical practice."[11] Brian Olshansky, director of cardiac electrophysiology at University of Iowa Hospitals and Larry Dossey, executive editor of *Alternative Therapies in Health and Medicine*, reflected in *The BMJ* on Leibovici's study: "Rather than dismissing studies of prayer because they do not make sense or confirm our existing knowledge, we should consider them seriously exactly for this reason. In the history of science, findings that do not fit in often yield the most profound breakthroughs."[12]

Going Chakra

In the early 2000's a team of fifteen M.D.'s and Ph.D.'s led by Duke's Mitchell Krucoff carried out the MANTRA (monitoring and actu-alization of noetic training) study. In addition to prayer it included what the researchers call music, imagery and touch (MIT) therapy. This involves giving patients healing touches via the Hindu-influ-enced "chakra connection" technique. The imagery component involved having the patient form mental images of peaceful and relaxing places. No description was given for the music component. There were 748 coronary care patients divided into four groups, located at nine medical centers. One group had MIT therapy only, one group prayer only, one group MIT and prayer, and a control group had standard care. The intercessors were Christians, Muslims, Jews, and Buddhists. No one patient group recovered faster than any other group. However, the mortality rate was slightly lower for those assigned both prayer and MIT therapy and for those assigned MIT only, versus those assigned prayer only or those assigned standard care.[13]

Prior to the main study they carried out a feasibility pilot study. The only difference in treatment was that stress relaxation techniques were used instead of music therapy. In this pilot study, patients assigned standard care had the lowest mortality rates, and the prayer-only group the second-lowest mortality. But the standard-care patients had higher complication rates compared with patients in all of the other groups. There were 25 to 30 percent fewer adverse outcomes in non-standard patients. And of those groups, the prayer-only patients had the lowest short-term and long-term complication rates. The intercessors consisted of Protestant, Catholic, Jewish, Buddhist, and New Age groups located in the United States and abroad.[14]

An Australian writer pointed to concerns about de-personalizing prayer through scientific studies, and called to mind theologian N.T. Wright's quote, "Prayer is not a penny in the slot machine. You can't just put in a coin and get out a chocolate bar." Nevertheless, he went through twenty-one intercessory prayer studies published between 1964 and 2011. Fourteen of them revealed a positive and statistically significant health effect. Seven found no effect. He summed it up this way: "With about two-thirds of the studies and reviews indicating that prayer assists healing, it is hard to deny that something is happening."[15]

Chapter 14

CAVEATS TO CONSIDER

The research shows overwhelmingly positive health and wellness effects of active worship. What about negative effects? In an area as large and varied as religion and health, inevitably there will be areas of concern. Are there instances in which religion can hamper physical or psychological well-being? Sometimes yes, when practiced incorrectly.

We've discussed ways in which religious devotees cope with difficult life challenges. But sometimes there's the mentality of totally relying on divine intervention to resolve issues rather than taking action oneself. It could lead to neglect of diet, exercise, or medicines, thus impeding recovery.[1] Or an ill person could resist proven medical treatments in favor of perceived faith-based treatments.[2] Instead, the faithful should take action themselves to the extent possible while still trusting in God.

As described by Christina Rush and colleagues at CU Denver, forms of religious coping include: 1) Collaborative, in which the attitude is shared responsibility with God, i.e. "God and I are in this together. God will do His part and I'll do mine"; 2) Deferred, a passive approach in which "It's all in God's hands and out of my control"; 3) Abandoned, where the person feels abandoned by God and fully responsible for his or her own health problems, i.e. "I'm on my own because God has abandoned me"; and 4) Self-Directed, involving no thought of God or a higher power — "I'll take care of this myself. I don't believe in God." Of the four, studies reveal the Collaborative approach elicits the best physical and mental health. Self-Directed has mixed outcomes, Deferred generally has negative results, and Abandoned has the strongest negative outcomes.[3] So attitude is important.

The Abandoned mindset connotes anger with God. Or they're angry with themselves, thinking the illness or injury is a type of divine punishment. They may have feelings of guilt, shame, and negative self-worth. Such negative religious coping or "religious struggle" is associated with slower recovery, higher mortality, and greater anxiety. With survey data from about 600 patients, Bowling Green State's Kenneth Pargament and colleagues disclosed that those who considered God as punishing or abandoning them had a death rate during the next two years up to 30 percent higher than the other patients.[4] The scholars recommend that in these situations doctors should consider referring patients to clergy.[5] It's essential to look to the Judeo-Christian teachings of repentance, mercy, and forgiveness to overcome feelings of guilt and shame. It's not enough just to have faith in God. The right kind of faith is key—knowing God is full of justice yet mercy, omnipresent yet intimate.

Another misuse of religion is wishing divine vengeance on someone. This not only violates the principle of forgiveness but also shows malice. Other pitfalls include: putting off important decisions in the hope of receiving a sign from God; excessive guilt and disproportionate acts of penance to atone for perceived misdeeds; spending all of one's time on worship to the neglect of one's spouse and at-home children, especially to the neglect of their spiritual health; blind allegiance to charismatic self-proclaimed religious leaders who have sinister agendas (such as the notorious Jim Jones or David Koresh); blaming one's bad behavior on malevolent forces; and scrupulosity, which entails fearing one has sinned when one hasn't.[6]

Mental illness, not religiosity itself, can drive many of these behaviors. The healthy practice of religion is key. "Mature employments of religion that emphasize love, forgiveness, acceptance, mercy and compassion are difficult to neuroticize," writes Koenig.[7]

Simon Dein of University College London, while pointing out that religious practice generally is conducive to mental health, cautions that "excessive reliance on ritual and prayer may delay seeking psychiatric help and consequently worsen prognosis." This is certainly possible; a person comfortable in one's faith should be able to recognize when it's time to seek a mental health professional. Dein also writes of "excessive devotion to religious practice that can result in a family breakup," and that "differences in the level of religiosity between spouses can result in marital disharmony."[8] This also is true. When both spouses start out nonreligious and one becomes religious, the other may be quite upset over it. A famous conversion story involves former *Chicago Tribune* investigative reporter Lee Strobel who as an atheist was mortified when his wife became Christian. He almost was ready to divorce over it. Fortunately that never happened. He launched what turned out to be an almost two-year investigation into Christianity with the intention of proving to her it's based on a false premise. By the end of his investigation he concluded that the startling claims of this belief system are true after all. So he became a Christian himself.[9] But what if he hadn't investigated Christianity and instead stuck to his atheism? To be sure, the risk of marital problems should be no disincentive to embrace faith. That would be putting the world before God, which Christianity teaches against. And besides, when one spouse sincerely embraces God, He usually ensures the marital relationship works out, just as it did for the Strobels.

Dein also warns "religion can promote rigid thinking, overdependence on laws and rules, an emphasis on guilt and sin, and disregard for personal individuality and autonomy." Some of these actually can be positives. It's precisely the laws and rules of God that benefit a person. Churchgoing involves behaving in a way God wants us to behave according to teachings found in sacred scripture. Call them what you will—laws, rules, precepts, exhortations, promptings, tenets, or teachings; time after time it has been found that those who adhere to such teachings are on the whole healthier, happier, and more successful in life. In the same way, abiding by laws and rules imposed by civil society, like stopping at red lights, is a good thing.

"Rigid thinking" often is construed as following precepts of a belief system that may not reflect the prevailing sentiment in secular society. Take the Ten Commandments. Apart from thou shalt not kill and thou shalt not steal, the rest of the Commandments are perfectly legal according to civil law—and killing is even legal as long as the person is pre-born. Some may consider it rigid to abide by all of the Commandments such as attending church every Sunday, avoiding saying "Oh my God" when not praying, avoiding adultery and fornication, and eschewing abortion. Instead of the pejorative "rigid," better words would be conscientious, observant, scrupulous, self-disciplined, resolute, law-abiding, faithful, dutiful, or compliant. Faithfully following God's laws actually brings joy.

> "If you keep my commandments, you will abide in my love, just as I have kept my Father's commandments and abide in His love. I have said these things to you so that my joy may be in you, and that your joy may be complete." (John 15:10-11)

An emphasis on guilt and sin isn't always bad either. Without it, people wouldn't think they're doing anything wrong and continue to indulge in whatever vices they please—whether it be drinking, smoking, lying, cheating, or sleeping around. People *should* feel guilty and remorseful for bad behavior. Sometimes it's only a religious institution that ever brings that to their attention. Dein also mentions a "disregard for personal individuality and autonomy."[10] If that means deciding against engaging in behaviors that are sinful according to one's religion, such as those mentioned above, then it may very well turn out to be a good thing for the individual's overall well-being.

When Sanctification Gets Tested

Chapters 6 and 7 discuss family relationships being looked upon as sanctified and blessed by God, whether it be a marriage, parent-child, sibling-sibling, or other relationship. This fosters stronger bonds, greater forgiveness, less conflict, and greater marital and parent-child satisfaction. However, when conflicts are so large or when efforts to prevent them fall short, there may be costs to sanctification. Individuals could have unrealistic expectations and assume sanctified bonds are just that—sacrosanct and immune to injury. Stressful and/or unexpected life events inevitably arise such as job layoffs, serious illnesses, or adolescent rebellion. Relations could sour, defying expectations that sanctification will stave off such developments. That could prompt someone to believe he has failed spiritually or that God has failed him, exacerbating an already difficult situation and generating stronger negative emotions than would otherwise be the case. Bowling Green State's Mahoney and colleagues give an example. "When couples who sanctify childrearing discover that their personal and marital adjustment to parenting is more difficult than anticipated, they may feel more anxious, guilt-ridden, or upset." They could have unrealistic expectations and lack skills to resolve conflict. After a couple gets married, for example, they may acknowledge marriage can be difficult yet place so much confidence in sanctification that they fail to take concrete and necessary steps to better prepare themselves for the future. They may have certain expectations for family life but be unable to handle the conflicts.

A new mother may think of her role as sanctified but be hit with postpartum depression, and be unable or refuse to deal with the condition. Another instance is when someone violates a rule of moral behavior as laid out by one's religious tradition. The result could be guilt, anxiety, defensiveness, and psychological distress that are more intense than if the same behavior took place under no sanctification. (This often happens with porn.[11]) The emotions may make the person reluctant to even disclose the wrongdoing to other family members and thus prolong the secret, causing even more guilt and distress, and exacerbating the pain of the others when the secret is finally exposed. Another risk is that, because family members wish to protect sanctified relationships at all costs, they're more tolerant of wrongdoing or mistreatment than they would be under non-sanctification.

While consequences of breaches of accepted modes of behavior can be more intense under sanctification, religious traditions have methods to ameliorate the fallout or heal damaged relationships. In the case of marital infidelity the injured party may forgive the unfaithful spouse and help rebuild things. There also are rituals enabling repentance and reconciliation, such as the sacrament of confession in which a priest prescribes penance in the form of prayers or actions to atone for the misdeeds.

Sanctified relationships may come with certain preconceived notions about what such a relationship should entail. One person's notion could differ from another's. For example they could have conflicting ideas on gender roles. Such disagreements may be especially intractable because they relate to strongly held spiritual beliefs. "The inability of family members to be flexible and transform their assumptions underlying the nature of sanctified relationships may increase maladaptive communication methods (e.g., arguing, blaming), emotional distance within dyads, and subtle or overt rejection from the family," write Mahoney and colleagues.[12]

In the case of divorce, parties who considered the union as sanctified—whether it be one or both spouses, the children, or parents of the divorcing couple—may feel a profound sense of spiritual failure, guilt, and bewilderment over the separation of something they thought God joined together. They may consider the most sanctified institution of their lives as shattered, and feel removed from God. As one woman observed, "Equating the union of marriage with the union with God can be devastating for people going through a divorce. If the marriage has been a metaphor for union with God, then the obvious sequel is that the divorce symbolizes separation from God. The broken relationship with spouse is experienced as a broken relationship with God." One or both divorcees may feel they don't deserve the presence of God and perhaps stop attending church.[13] Such attitudes of course are misguided, neglecting God's abundant mercy.

Mahoney and colleagues reiterate that "sanctification appears to be a protective factor in non-distressed samples."[14] In other words, sanctification strengthens relationships and helps prevent them from souring. But inevitably in life, distress sometimes sets in.

Christianity teaches life isn't a bowl of cherries—and that there's no guarantee being devoutly religious will steer you clear of pain and suffering. It's those situations that test one's faith. Sanctification can help you cope in this regard—minus the prideful attitude of "I'm so holy nothing can happen to me." The key is to pass the test, pick yourself up, and carry on. As Pope Benedict XVI is reported to have said, "You were not made for comfort. You were made for greatness."

Religious Rivalries

Another downside are inter-group resentments. Humans seemingly have an innate tendency to treat outgroups with hostility or regard them as inferior, whether it involves tribes, ethnic groups, language groups, nationalities, political parties, sports-team fandom, religions, or religious denominations. Examples of the latter are Catholic-Protestant rivalries and past wars. There also are the Muslim-Jewish conflicts, Sunni-Shiite rivalries, and perhaps most shameful, the pogroms and genocide against Jews by those purporting to be Christian—although the worst perpetrators in the National Socialist leadership had long prior abandoned their Christianity and instead embraced occult beliefs and practices.[15]

Negative ingroup/outgroup attitudes are harmful mentally, physically, and spiritually. Someone harboring anger and resentment toward those of another denomination, religion, or non-religion not only hurts himself psychologically but also physically owing to those molecules of emotion discussed in chapter 2. He hurts himself spiritually because he's sinning. His attitude of superiority is the sin of pride—widely considered to be the worst of the Seven Deadly Sins. Jesus taught humility. The Lord also warned against anger and was particularly emphatic against unforgiveness (e.g., Matthew 18:23-35). Of course, when resentments boil over into insults, slander, and violence, the sins rise to whole new levels.

Disagreements between religions and religious denominations should be handled with courtesy and respect. Differing opinions above all should stem from love, i.e. the desire to help others secure eternal salvation—through rational persuasion, discussion, and example.

To be sure, the nonreligious certainly aren't exempt from such ingroup-outgroup animosity. Atheists have committed some of the worst crimes against humanity, targeting people of faith in such places as the Soviet Union, Cuba, China, North Korea, and Eastern Europe*. And on a less-ferocious level, even today in the world's advanced democracies, nonbelievers often scorn believers. In fact, in America the main rivalry has moved from a largely Protestant vs. Catholic one in days of old, to a largely atheist/agnostic vs. religious one. Given the intense secularization of society and spread of atheism and agnosticism, devout Protestants, Catholics, and (mainly Orthodox) Jews are more allies than rivals, especially in the political sphere.

---

* See, for example, Rev. Richard Wurmbrand's *Tortured for Christ*, depicting atrocities he and many others endured in Romanian prisons solely because of their Christian faith.

Chapter 15

RELIGION AND YOUR DOCTOR

After being an emergency room physician for nineteen years, Bruce Feldstein is a chaplain at Stanford University Medical Center and professor at the medical school. One of the things prompting his change of role was an experience he had while a doctor. Upon informing an eighty-six year-old she had brain cancer, she reacted with devastation, calling it a "death sentence." Moved with sympathy, and seeing she wore a cross necklace, Feldstein offered to pray with her. So he put her Christian hands in his Jewish hands and they prayed, while a Stanford intern looked on in disbelief. Afterward the woman was much calmer and thanked Dr. Feldstein for his consideration. "Patients are suffering, truly suffering, as a result of illness," lamented Feldstein. "They're lonely, they're scared, they're terrified. These are existential issues; these are spiritual issues." Feldstein helped launch a course at Stanford for medical students titled "Spirituality and Meaning in Medicine."[1]

Another story, told by Harold Koenig, involves a patient with a quite different attitude. While attending a funeral one winter, Mrs. Bernard slipped on the ice and fell, fracturing her hip. In the hospital, the pain of that injury was enough to deal with, but things got worse when she was stricken with a bad lung infection. Her stay there extended to a month. She had other things on her mind as well: the funeral she attended was her husband's. He suffered a fatal stroke, leaving her alone in a large city. Only months prior to that, she lost her only son in a car accident. When she was ready to be discharged, the surgeon was concerned about her emotional state and asked Dr. Koenig to check on her. When he walked in she said, "Hello! Dr. Jones said you'd be by today. Come sit down." Putting down her Bible she asked, "What can I do for you, doctor?" She seemed strangely at peace, mentioning that she still had a daughter in Tennessee and eventually would be moving closer to her. Dr. Koenig initially thought she was in denial. But after chatting at length, he thrust that idea aside. After mentioning how well she seemed to be holding up, he asked her, "What's your secret? How do you cope the way you do?" After a momentary silence, with Bible in hand, she smiled. "This is what helps me. Whenever I get to feeling sad or blue, I pick up my Bible and begin reading it, and somehow this calms me." She continued, "When I wake up at night and feel alone or afraid, I read my Bible or talk to God."[2]

She wasn't Dr. Koenig's only patient who said their faith helps them through infirmities. It got him curious, prompting him to search for academic studies on this topic. At that time, in the early 1980s, there nary was one to be found. So he started conducting studies of his own.[3] Around that same time, as a graduate student in public health at UNC, Jeff Levin happened upon several obscure studies finding a positive effect of churchgoing on cardiovascular health. Intrigued, during the course of the next few years he uncovered over two hundred studies pertaining to the religion-health relationship, dating to the nineteenth century. "Although these studies had been done and their results published, apparently almost no one knew they existed," recounted Levin in his book *Religion and Medicine: A History of the Encounter Between Humanity's Two Greatest Institutions*. "I felt like an explorer who had made a startling discovery." In 1987 he wrote a review of his research published in the *Journal of Religion and Health*. The same year other researchers, working independently, did the same. ("There must have been something in the water that year," he quipped.)[4]

Thus began what eventually was to become an avalanche of scholarly research on the topic. The publication of hundreds of studies in the 1990s confirmed a positive relationship between religion and both physical and mental health, followed by an explosion of such studies since then, now to the tune of more than 6,000.[5] Studies by Koenig, Levin, Ellen Idler, Robert Hummer, and many others helped dispel the notion within the scientific community that religious belief and practice are minor or irrelevant in influencing health and longevity. As discussed in chapter 1, Hummer's rigorous study published in 1999 ascertained that regular churchgoers live six to seven years longer on average. In 2001, Koenig, Michael McCullough, and David Larson published the first edition of the *Handbook of Religion and Health*. These developments prompted many health professionals to sit up and take notice. Whereas only a handful of America's medical schools offered courses related to spirituality and medicine in the mid-1990s, now nearly all of them do (albeit most of them are elective rather than required courses[6]), largely due to increased interest from patients as well as greater openness on the part of doctors to address such issues. Even the Association of American Medical Colleges has recommendations and guidance regarding spirituality.[7]

On the mental side, the modern-day history of the association between religion and psychiatry has been more colorful and almost has come full circle. Until the 1800s religious institutions largely were responsible for caring for the mentally ill. Then during the latter part of that century the French psychiatrist Jean-Martin Charcot and his pupil Sigmund Freud had a profound effect on the direction of psychiatry. Both were said to be atheists, vigorously integrating their anti-religious views into their field. Charcot associated religion with irrationality and neurosis, as did Freud.[8] But sometimes even Freud spoke positively about religion's effect on mental health. Recognizing the value of having a sense of meaning and purpose, Freud admitted religion engenders that. Surprisingly, considering how hostile he seemed toward religion in other writings, Freud wrote in *Civilization and Its Discontents*, "Once again, only religion can answer the question of the purpose of life. One can hardly be wrong in concluding that the idea of life having a purpose stands and falls with the religious system." Elsewhere, in a letter to Swiss Lutheran minister and lay psychoanalyst Oskar Pfister and also while addressing the Vienna Psychoanalytic Society, he stated that faith may help ward off neuroses, recognizing the "extraordinary increase in neuroses since the power of religions has waned."[9] (History now repeats itself.)

Nevertheless, for about a century until the 1990s, the hostile attitude toward religion was widespread among psychiatrists, who generally are less religious than their patients, if not atheistic. Practitioners typically viewed the religiosity of patients as irrelevant and unimportant at best, delusional at worst. "The suggestion that religion might influence mental or physical health outcomes was greeted with skepticism and even hostility by many medical researchers, and it evoked images of faith healers and charlatans among the general public," write Ellison and Levin.[10]

Carl Jung was a notable exception, observing in 1932 that the absence of religion was at the crux of the problem for patients in their thirties and above, "having lost that which living religions of every age have given to their believers." He later wrote that "neurosis must be understood as the suffering of a human being who has not discovered what life means for him."[11] Holocaust survivor and prominent psychiatrist Viktor Frankl echoed Jung's sentiments, saying the notion of serving a higher power and fulfilling a higher purpose is of "enormous psychotherapeutic and psychohygienic value."[12]

Notwithstanding Jung and Frankl, the bias was evident in the American Psychiatric Association's *Diagnostic and Statistical Manual of Mental Disorders*, the standard reference manual for the classification of mental illnesses. Patrick Fagan reports that the third edition of the manual brought up religious examples in a negative light, associating them with delusions and incoherence. But the subsequent edition published in 1994 corrected that bias. A few years prior, anti-religious bias in the Minnesota Multiphasic Personality Inventory, a widely used psychological test, was removed.[13] The correction reflected a recognition in the psychology field that religion actually improves mental health.

"Support of the patient's spirituality has been deemed an ethical imperative, reflecting a physician's commitment to the patient's best interest," write Kanita Dervic and her Columbia colleagues in a study published in the *American Journal of Psychiatry*.[14] Religion-based therapy has seen faster recovery from depression compared with standard secular cognitive-behavioral therapy. In 1994 a category was introduced into the *Diagnostic and Statistical Manual*: "Religious or Spiritual Problems." Later the APA issued guidelines on handling conflicts between psychiatrists' personal religious beliefs and psychiatric practice. And the Accreditation Council for Graduate Medical Education in its psychiatric training includes instruction on religion in psychiatric care.[15]

Interest in the positive impact of religion on mental health grew markedly in the 1990s. Ellison and Levin point to many factors behind it including:

- church-induced self-discipline in lifestyle and healthy behaviors.
- the social ties and formal and informal social support one gets through church.
- positive self-perceptions.
- religious-based coping mechanisms.
- positive emotions such as love and forgiveness.
- healthy beliefs such as hope and optimism. And interestingly,
- "hypothesized mechanisms, such as the existence of a healing bioenergy."[16]

The change of attitude in the psychiatry field was evident in the works of prominent psychologist Albert Ellis (1913-2007), pioneer of rational emotive behavior therapy (REBT) and outspoken atheist. For most of his career he considered religion to contribute to psychological distress and in 1980 even published a pamphlet titled "The Case Against Religiosity." Later in life he substantially toned down his rhetoric, acknowledging faith in God can be psychologically healthy. He even co-authored a book with two religious psychologists on integrating religion with REBT.[17]

As with religion and physical health, during the 1990s and especially after the turn of the century, study after study came out on religion and mental health, the vast majority of them showing a positive relationship.[18] The psychiatry profession took notice. Writing in 2010, Simon Dein of University College London reported that at least 50 percent of psychiatrists considered it appropriate to inquire about patients' religious lives. Religion is recognized as a significant enough factor in the psychiatry field that practitioners are often trained in how to ask patients about their spirituality. They are directed to be sensitive to the patient's religious views and be as neutral as possible without manipulating or influencing those views. Dein notes that recommending prayer or other direct religious interventions remains controversial in psychiatry[19]—which isn't surprising considering the number of secularists in that field.

So there's still a long way to go. Even though 84 percent of the world's population is religiously affiliated and most of the rest believe in God or a higher power, even though four out of five people afflicted with serious mental illness use religion to cope, even though abundant research shows religion/spirituality is associated with less mental illness and greater happiness, the stark reality is that "no other social phenomenon so widespread is ignored by academic psychiatrists," states *Crossroads*, echoing an article by David Rosmarin of Harvard along with Kenneth Pargament at Bowling Green State and Harold Koenig at Duke. "Why ignore this potentially therapeutic element in mental health care?" Nevertheless, there's hope. Their 2020 article appeared in *Lancet Psychiatry*, one of the top mainstream psychiatry journals in the world. As noted in *Crossroads*, "The mere fact that the editors of this journal are willing to publish an article like this reflects the growing acknowledgement that religion/spirituality can have a significant impact on mental health, thus deserving the attention of mental health professionals."[20]

Seeking Spiritual Care

Religious therapy can outperform standard secular therapy, with faster recovery times. Lewis and Clark College's Rebecca Propst and colleagues looked at the effectiveness of religious therapy on depression. In the study were fifty-nine religious patients with nonpsychotic, nonbipolar depression. A portion of them were given cognitive behavioral therapy with religious content. Another portion had no religious content. The third subset of patients had pastoral counseling, which involved listening to and discussing Bible verses. The results: both the religious content therapy and pastoral counseling groups had lower post-treatment depression, compared with the nonreligious content subgroup. One surprise was that religious-content patients treated by nonreligious therapists enjoyed superior results than patients treated by religious therapists.[21] In another study, 100 percent of patients in the religious group achieved their goals compared with 57 percent in the nonreligious group.[22]

Citing several studies, VanderWeele indicates that integrating religion into therapy—including forgiveness therapy—can result in higher recovery rates than purely secular therapy, but not always. In general, spiritual care often benefits both the mentally and physically ill. Not only do patients usually desire it, but it's associated with lower costs and less-aggressive treatment. In the study finding a five-fold lower suicide rate among women who attend church at least weekly (see chapter 10), VanderWeele and his colleagues write, "For patients who are already religious, service attendance might be encouraged as a form of meaningful social participation. Religion and spirituality may be an underappreciated resource that psychiatrists and clinicians could explore with their patients, as appropriate."[23]

For both psychological and physical treatment, proponents of spiritual care say a physician merely has to administer a brief spiritual history; if the patient isn't religious, any discussion of spiritual care quickly can be dropped.[*] A doctor reported that in his sixteen years of practice, no patients with incurable or fatal illnesses ever responded negatively to his inquiries about their spiritual lives—and that such enquiries often were helpful.[24] A survey of patients carried out by Andrew Newberg and colleagues at UPenn showed

---

[*] "Simply recording the patient's religious denomination and whether they want to see a chaplain, the procedure in most hospitals today, is NOT taking a spiritual history," notes Koenig in "Religion, Spirituality, and Health: The Research and Clinical Implications," *ISRN Psychiatry*, Dec. 2012.

that some 70 percent of patients wanted their physicians to ask about their spiritual and religious beliefs; surprisingly, even half of the nonreligious patients wanted that—perhaps because it at least would convey that the doctor cares about them as a person. But still, "It's not like we can tell people, because they're sick, to go home, take two prayers and call us in the morning," remarked Newberg. "Therefore we have to be very cautious about how religious and spiritual beliefs and practices are actually used in the context of health care."[25]

But often, prayers can be fine. When a religious patient was having panic attacks for fear of Covid-19, the attending physician not only prescribed clonazepam three times a day but also instructed the patient to recite aloud Psalm 91 after each dose. Multiple times it mentions protection from pestilence.[26]

There are other practical reasons for asking patients about their faith. For example a religion may prohibit certain medications or foods. Susan Stangl of UCLA told *Newsweek* about a Muslim patient who couldn't eat or drink during the day, presumably during the Ramadan fast. So she chose a medication that could be taken at night. Fortunately she asked the patient about his religious preferences— otherwise a daytime-only medicine would have posed a problem.[27]

Powell, Shahabi, and Thoresen in "Religion and Spirituality: Linkages to Physical Health" state that, given religious institutions' wide availability and low cost, church attendance "could be a very cost-effective way to maintain the health of elderly people with disability or chronic diseases." After all, it's cheaper than Lipitor (see chapter 1). In addition to helping to prevent illness, Powell et al. suggest it can be a coping resource for those who've taken ill. "Then it would support the recognition of spiritual counselors as an important part of the medical team." They add the caveat that this proposal has been met with considerable controversy.[28]

This isn't surprising. Opponents of spiritual care (which includes recommending religious activities such as church services) say it can cause tension and antagonism owing to differences in religious views between patients and physicians and/or lack of such training in physicians. Richard Sloan, director of behavioral medicine at Co-lumbia-Presbyterian Medical Center, is a critic of the role of religion in medicine. A paper he co-authored averred that physicians could overstep boundaries if they start "prescribing religion," and that reli-gion shouldn't be "intervened upon." Echoing what's in the previous chapter, he and his colleagues posited that associating religion with health might erroneously convey that the illness stems from religious or moral failure, as a type of divine punishment. "It's bad enough to be sick, it's worse still to be gravely ill, but to add to that the burden of remorse and guilt for some supposed failure of religious devotion is unconscionable," thundered Sloan in an interview with *Newsweek*.[29] Another concern is the patient relying too much on God and not enough on his or her own actions in improving health, such as exercising and eating healthy. Sloan et al. did, however, concede that discussion of religion may be appropriate when the doctor and patient share a common faith.[30]

Responding to Sloan's critique, Koenig acknowledged the ethical issues involved but argued that as a whole, the evidence is clear that religious practice positively impacts health.[31] He's pleased that medical schools are taking notice. "It is gratifying that medical pro-fessionals are at last coming to recognize that there is more to their patients than just physical bodies."[32] He also observed, "There are questions of meaning and purpose that science just doesn't have very good answers to. Also, patients want to be talked to. They are tired of being treated like bodies, just physical bodies."[33] As noted above, Koenig urges doctors to get spiritual histories, e.g. asking patients questions such as, "Is religion a source of comfort or stress?", "Do you have any religious beliefs that would influence decision-making?," and "Do you have any spiritual needs that someone should address?"[34] He says the majority of doctors are still reluctant to do this. "They're afraid to get into it, they don't want to argue with patients, they don't feel they're prepared or trained to do it, and so they just ignore it. But we're trying to push them to do it, and so I think the research is coming out to the point that many doctors are now doing it because they recognize it's important."[35]

Chapter 16

HEALTHY SELF AND CITIZENRY

"No other dimension of life in America—with the exception of stable marriages and families, which in turn are strongly tied to religious practice—does more to promote the well-being and soundness of the nation's civil society than citizens' religious observance," writes Patrick Fagan. "The widespread practice of religious beliefs is one of America's greatest national resources. It strengthens individuals, families, communities, and society as a whole. It significantly affects educational and job attainment and reduces the incidence of such major social problems as out-of-wedlock births, drug and alcohol addiction, crime, and delinquency."[1]

What responsible country would not want to alleviate social problems including crime, substance abuse, dropping out of school, incarceration, poor health, depression, anxiety, suicide, marital breakdown, porn addiction, and out-of-wedlock births? And what society would not want to raise the general level of mental and physical health, education, safety on the streets, revitalization of inner cities, school attendance, and charitable outreach? Church is one of the most effective ways to do that. Certainly, atheists and non-churchgoers can teach their children moral values and principles without the aid of religion. But religion has far more tools in that regard, starting with sacred scriptures.

One of the most visible benefits of religiosity is charitable giving. A nation in which most citizens donate and volunteer is a nation that's more just, equitable, and successful. Churchgoers do this more than non-churchgoers—89 percent versus 76 percent for money, and 82 percent versus 51 percent for volunteerism, according to a Gallup survey.[2] And that includes secular causes, not just religious ones.[3]

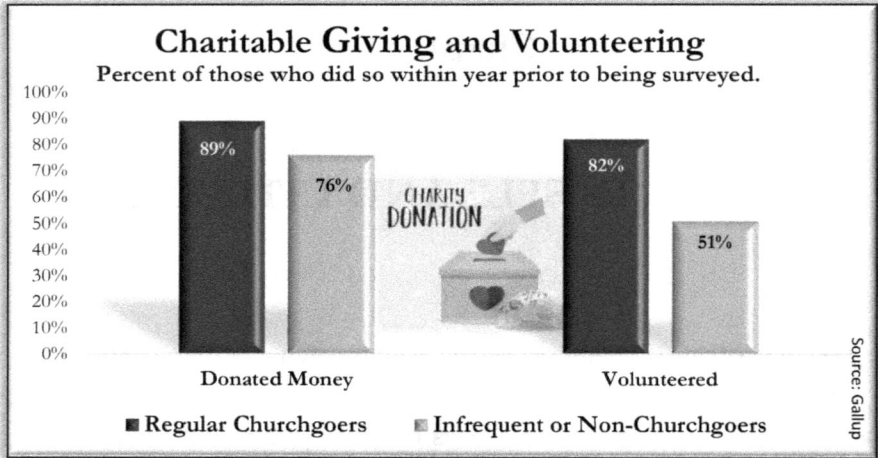

Charitable Giving and Volunteering
Percent of those who did so within year prior to being surveyed.

Donated Money — Regular Churchgoers 89%, Infrequent or Non-Churchgoers 76%
Volunteered — Regular Churchgoers 82%, Infrequent or Non-Churchgoers 51%

■ Regular Churchgoers   ▣ Infrequent or Non-Churchgoers

Source: Gallup

Benevolent Benefits

During these secular times, religion is often shunned and criti-cized. Many disagree with teachings against abortion, premarital sex, homosexual unions, and transgenderism. Those get all of the media attention. But they're just a tiny fraction of the precepts of a given religion. In Christianity, topics with scant media coverage are long-held moral and ethical teachings, most of which nearly every-one agrees are very good things—and that if they were practiced more often, the world would be a much better place. Following is a sampling of those teachings (with paraphrasing):

The Ten Commandments (Exodus 20:2-17 and Deuteronomy 5:6-21):
Love God with all your might, and shun false gods.
Honor the Sabbath day.
Don't take the Lord's name in vain.
Honor your father and mother.
Don't murder.
Don't commit adultery.
Don't steal.
Don't lie.
Don't covet anyone else's spouse.
Don't envy or covet anyone else's goods.

The Ten Commandments as summed up by Jesus Christ (Matthew 22:35-40, Mark 12:28-34, and Luke 10:27):
Love God with all of your heart, mind, and soul.
Love your neighbor as yourself.

The Corporal Works of Mercy (Matthew 25:31-46):
Give food, drink, clothing, and shelter to the poor.
Visit the sick.
Visit the imprisoned.
Bury the dead. (This originally applied to poor societies and dire situations when people literally died in the streets.)

The Spiritual Works of Mercy (various passages throughout the Bible):
Comfort the grief-stricken.
Practice forgiveness.
Bear wrongs patiently. (E.g., don't respond to hostility with hostility.)
Instruct the ignorant. (Teach people about the faith.)
Counsel the doubtful. (Help those struggling in their faith.)
Admonish sinners. (Gently let people know when they're choosing wrong.)
Comfort the afflicted.
Pray for the living and the dead.

The Beatitudes (Matthew 5:1-12):
Empathize with the poor by forgoing comforts from time to time — be "poor in spirit."
Have hope and courage during times of mourning.
Be humble.
Promote righteousness.
Be merciful.
Have a pure heart.
Promote peace.
Have hope and courage in the face of persecution.
Persevere in the face of scorn, slander, ridicule, or persecution.

Seven Deadly Sins (various Bible passages):
Avoid pride (i.e. arrogance/vanity), envy, greed, gluttony, laziness, lust, and anger.

Seven Cardinal Virtues (various Bible passages):
Have hope.
Have faith.
Practice love and charity.
Be prudent.
Practice justice.
Show fortitude.
Practice temperance/moderation when consuming food, alcohol, entertainment activities, and the like.

Fruits of the Holy Spirit (Galatians 5:22-23):
Charity, joy, peace, patience, kindness, goodness, generosity, gentleness, faithfulness, modesty, self-control, and chastity.

Can anyone deny that if everyone abided by all or most of the above, the world would be a much better place? What other institution promotes so many virtues and denounces so many vices?

Because it involves answering to a higher power, religion promotes morals and ethics within society in ways secular institutions cannot. The ultimate aim is to love God and become united with Him, which is carried out not only by worshipping Him but also by behaving morally and ethically. Because sin and evil essentially are manifestations of rebellion against God, the aim is to shun these so as to please God in this life and be with Him in the next.

One could point out that some religious leaders and practitioners don't live out their own religion's virtues and instead engage in high-profile vice. But it's the religion and its teachings that one should embrace, not some weak-kneed miscreants who claim leadership or membership in that religion yet fail miserably in practicing it themselves. Besides, it's said that Christianity is a hospital for sinners, not a sanctuary for saints. You can't realistically expect all or even most of its members to embody living sainthood.

It Pays to Be Nice

One of the biggest manifestations of a good and just society are the simple, everyday acts of kindness people carry out whether it be in the home, on the streets, at the workplace, at school, the store, or anywhere else. There are plenty of warm, friendly, and nice non-churchgoers. But Harvard's Robert Putnam and Notre Dame's David Campbell conclude that religious folks have the upper hand in that regard. In their book *American Grace*, which reports on the findings of their survey of more than 3,000 people, Putnam and Campbell disclose that the religious are "in some respects simply 'nicer'" in matters of everyday life. They are more likely to do such things as:

- give up their seat to a stranger.
- carry items for a stranger.
- give money to panhandlers.
- help an elderly neighbor with chores.
- let someone cut in front of them.
- lend money and items.
- give directions to someone on the street.
- care for pets or plants for someone who's away.

In addition to good neighborliness, the pious generally are more trusting. The authors write, "Religious Americans express significantly more trust than secular Americans do in shop clerks, people of their own ethnicity, people of other ethnicities, and even strangers. In short, religious people are both more trusting of virtually everyone else and (in the eyes of others) more trustworthy themselves."[4]

The strongest predictor of the extent to which someone is empathetic and altruistic isn't education, age, income, gender, or other demographic or ideological characteristic. It's religiosity. In Putnam and Campbell's survey, religious Americans scored significantly higher than nonreligious on an index of empathy and altruism. They much more commonly strongly agreed with such statements as, "Personally assisting people in trouble is very important to me." This empathy and altruism evoke generosity with time and money.

An earlier study carried out by S. Philip Morgan of UNC-Chapel Hill determined that regularly praying people aren't more likely than non-praying people to consider others to be fair, helpful, or trustworthy. However, echoing Putnam and Campbell's findings, Morgan found that churchgoers tend to be "nicer" overall. He analyzed National Opinion Research Center interviews of 1,467 adults, gauging their predisposition to being good, friendly, and cooperative. His study considered three prevailing narratives: (1) religious people are more intolerant and prejudiced, especially in light of harsh-sounding accounts of the Old Testament; (2) given the secularization of modern society, religious beliefs have a negligible effect on behavior and attitudes; and (3) religion engenders morality, humanitarianism, and "Golden Rule" behavior, especially in light of New Testament lessons emphasizing kindness, such as the Parable of the Good Samaritan.

Which narrative won out? You guessed it—the third. People who integrate prayer into their daily life by and large practice what they preach. They answered yes to the positives and no to the negatives to a much greater extent than those who seldom or never pray. Even the interviewers considered the prayerful interviewees to be more cooperative and friendly just based on the in-person interaction. Morgan pointed to another study that found the God-minded to be more likely to loan funds to a friend in need or give bus fare to a stranger. "Are religious people nice people?," he writes. "The answer seems to be yes—prayerful people do seem more friendly and cooperative."[5] And that goes hand-in-hand with being happy and healthy.

What is it about churchgoers that makes them nicer? It's church-going itself, declare Putnam and Campbell. "Church attendance itself seems to contain the secret ingredient in explaining why religious people are better, more trusting friends and neighbors." Someone of strong religious faith who rarely or never attends church, say the authors, is less likely to volunteer at a soup kitchen than an atheist actively involved in church (who, for example, may be there because of a spouse). The main driver of this generosity, they assert, is the social aspect of church—the friends made and groups attended there.

Even high-faith churchgoers who shun social interaction at church aren't much more neighborly than non-churchgoers, conclude Putnam and Campbell. It's religious belonging that matters, not so much religious believing. It's reasonable to expect theological teachings to prompt good neighborliness, but they surprisingly find no evidence of this in their survey. "What counts is not how well you learned the catechism or the Golden Rule as a child, but how involved you are nowadays in religious networks, as marked (for example) by churchgoing."[6]

This survey finding is curious. Based on clear teachings of Jesus in the Bible, Christians are called to do good works including the Corporal Works of Mercy listed above. Jesus declared that in the final reckoning, those who carry out these works, i.e. "the sheep," will be separated from "the goats"—and the goats end up in a place you don't want to go. That's a potent reason to be a good neighbor.

Why didn't this show up in the survey data? Campbell said there could be some other unmeasured factor that drives civic activity, but uncovering it would require a type of randomized experiment that would be impossible to set up. Nevertheless, he speculated that the driver of religious persons' civic activity is their co-religionist friends. "It may be the case that beliefs matter, but only when they are reinforced through one's friends," remarked Campbell. "Requests to contribute to a cause likely carry more weight when they come from someone who shares one's views, especially when those views are reinforced through scripture (for religious people) or other writings on ethics (for secular people). In other words, it is likely that the teachings matter, but when reinforced through a social network—which actually makes sense, as behavioral norms in general are also inculcated through social interactions."[7]

Advancing Agreeableness

As recounted two chapters ago, when Lee Strobel's wife broke the news she was a Bible believer, the *Chicago Tribune* investigative reporter and then-atheist was shocked. "My biggest fear with Leslie was that she was going to turn into some religious prude or something, and I thought nothing good could come out of this." But after a while, Lee began seeing positive changes in her character and values, and in the way she related to him and their children. "I was pleasantly surprised—even fascinated—by the fundamental changes in her character, her integrity, and her personal confidence." As for Lee, when he finally embraced Jesus after seeing the historical evidence for his resurrection (the linchpin confirming Jesus's claim to be the Son of God), a similar transformation happened in him. No longer was he the "profane, angry, verbally harsh, and all too often absent" father to whom his five-year-old daughter was so accustomed. She duly noticed the change in him, telling her mom, "Mommy, I want God to do for me what he's done for Daddy."[8]

No guarantees of course, but church can do those things to a spouse. Research confirms it. Survey respondents who participate in religious activities and devote attention to their spiritual life also place high value on relationship, social, and civic goals. They include having a satisfying spousal relationship, having harmonious relationships with parents and siblings, and working to promote others' welfare.[9] It's always better to be around a sweetie than a sourpuss.

Psychologists have identified what they call the Big Five dimensions of personality. These consistently manifest themselves in interviews, observations, and self-descriptions, in a wide array of people from a variety of cultures. They are: Openness, Conscientiousness, Extraversion, Agreeableness, and Neuroticism. McCullough and Willoughby report that traits most closely associated with religiousness are Agreeableness and Conscientiousness. These facilitate one's ability to conform to the wishes and feelings of others. Conscientiousness is the state of being careful, diligent, and scrupulous about performing tasks, and taking seriously their obligations. Agreeableness reflects a desire for social harmony and getting along. It values considerateness, kindness, generosity, trust, helpfulness, and willingness (to an extent) to sacrifice or compromise one's interests for the benefit of others. Agreeable people tend to be optimistic about human nature.[10] Who wouldn't want those traits in a spouse?

Mind you, a study disclosed that religiousness may discourage the pursuit of goals related to independence and individuality. Another reported that religiousness is unrelated to the goals of pursuing wealth, producing artistic work, having new and different experiences, and having fun.[11] But we all know that holy rollers would never turn down good, clean, wholesome fun.

Primed for Generosity

To better determine if religious concepts lead to more altruistic, benevolent behavior—what social scientists call pro-social behavior—Azim Shariff and Ara Norenzayan of the psychology department at the University of British Columbia sought to activate such concepts in test subjects' minds implicitly, without having them consciously reflect on the concepts. As described in their paper "God Is Watching You" they conducted the study twice—using participants drawn from the UBC student body and then from greater Vancouver.

Shariff and Norenzayan primed half of their subjects with God concepts. They had them unscramble five sentences containing the target words spirit, divine, God, sacred, and prophet, so the end result would be phrases such as "she felt the spirit" or "the dessert was divine." The other half unscrambled five sentences containing neutral words unrelated to religion. Each participant started out with ten one-dollar coins and had the choice to keep or give away as many as he or she would like to an anonymous stranger. Previous demonstrations of the exercise without the God priming showed time and again the majority act selfishly, giving away little or nothing.

The investigators' tests confirmed that result. In their first study (with the college students) those with no God priming gave an average of $1.84, with 52 percent of them parting with $1 or less, and none giving away more than $5. By contrast, those primed with God concepts donated an average of $4.22. That's almost two-and-a-half times as much as the non-God-primed subjects. Sixty-four percent of them left $5 or more.

Here's an interesting twist: there were atheists as well as believers. So a question is, would God concepts motivate atheists to act more benevolent even though they ostensibly don't believe in God? It turned out that even for them, God concepts boosted generosity.

In the second study with residents of greater Vancouver, Shariff and Norenzayan made a few modifications, including priming them with secular concepts of justice: civic, jury, court, police, and contract. They replicated the main findings from the first study. And interestingly, the effect of the law enforcement prime was almost as large as the religious prime. So implicit activation of secular concepts of law and justice curbs selfishness as well.[12]

Atheists Extol Religion

The French philosopher Voltaire (1694-1778) generally was against organized religion, at least as it applied to himself. It's said he nevertheless insisted that none of his friends or associates discuss atheism in the presence of his servants. "I want my lawyer, tailor, valets, even my wife, to believe in God," he said. "I think that if they do, I shall be robbed less and cheated less."[13]

Voltaire recognized the societal advantages of religion. So many modern-day atheists echo these sentiments that, as discussed in chapter 5, even Richard Dawkins has significantly toned down his rhetoric, finally admitting that belief in God can benefit society.

Other atheists speak even more highly of it. When first presented with the claim that religion improves mental health, Bruce Sheiman, author of *An Atheist Defends Religion*, defiantly denied it. But then he looked at the evidence. He reviewed a meta-analysis of hundreds of studies on the subject—covering all ages, many demographic groups, and spanning decades. It forced him to acknowledge that active worshippers are mentally, emotionally, and physically healthier. "The gold standard of atheistic evidence—empirical evidence—leaves few doubts that religion is good for the health of the individual and society as a whole." He also observes, "On balance, religion provides a combination of psychological, emotional, moral, communal, existential, and even physical-health benefits that no other institution can replicate." Atheism, he admits, is "an impoverished belief system."[14]

Alain de Botton, author of *Religion for Atheists*, argues that religions are instrumental in helping people better structure themselves and society. As the book title implies, de Botton is a non-believer. Yet he praises religion not only for its positive effect on human behavior but also for the rich cultural heritage associated with it. Without the support structures religion brings, he said, we'd be in a wasteland. "I like Christmas carols. I like the atmosphere of old churches. I like religious works of art. I like the idea of pilgrimage, fasting and feasting," he told an audience at a Canadian art gallery.[15] He urges nonbelievers and believers alike to look to religions for lessons in improving interpersonal relations, suppressing envy and other deadly sins, appreciating art, and building a sense of community, among other things. Though he evidently hasn't accepted religious doctrines (at least not yet; maybe he'll come around), he loves the art, music, and architecture associated with them. It's thanks to those doctrines that such objects of beauty sprang up.

Religious art and architecture aim to instill a sense of the transcendent, raising hearts and minds to God and heaven. Catholic author Michael S. Rose writes, "These elements—indeed the whole of the church edifice—must create an other-worldly feel that inspires man to worship God, to humble himself before his Creator, to partake in the sacred mysteries, and to focus himself on the eternal."[16]

The Prosperity Gospel

If religion teaches honesty, integrity, and trust, would it not follow that it promotes economic growth? In their zeal to spread the faith, religious missionaries spread books and literacy, technology and skills, and civic institutions. This fostered rising living standards. UT Austin sociologist Robert Woodberry writes that Protestants were particularly instrumental in this because of their emphasis on literacy in order to read the Bible.[17]

Developing countries often lack strong governmental enforcement mechanisms against corruption and wrongdoing. Widespread belief in spiritual enforcement mechanisms—i.e. temporal and/or eternal consequences for wrongdoing based on the teachings of one's religion—should not only reduce corruption but also, through engendering trust, facilitate trade and commerce. Robert Barro and his wife Rachel McCleary, both of the Harvard economics department, looked at this prospect. Their study included dozens of countries based on surveys asking about religious beliefs and practices, covering Christianity, Hinduism, Islam, and Buddhism. As predicted, religious commitment and involvement positively influence economic growth. Particularly interesting is that the more a given population believes in hell, the greater the economic growth—even when religious attendance stays flat. "There is also some indication that the stick represented by the fear of hell is more potent for growth than the carrot from the prospect of heaven," write the husband-wife team. They suggest religious beliefs enhance productivity through greater honesty, thrift, openness to strangers, and a stronger work ethic.[18] Paradoxically, they also found that developing countries with a high rate of religious service attendance tend to grow more slowly than those with lower attendance, perhaps due to greater consumption of resources by the church sector. But they seem to indicate this may not necessarily be the case if, within a given population, belief in hell and heaven rises with attendance.[19] It may also only appear that church attendance is associated with slower growth because as countries develop economically, religious practice tends to drop off.

In any event, in eighteenth-century Britain the Quakers became dominant in finance thanks in part to their reputation for honesty. Likewise in more recent times, Orthodox Jews have presided over the New York diamond trade. In such an endeavor involving highly valuable tiny commodities that easily can be stolen, it's crucial to maintain a high level of trust with commercial partners. Several studies have found that merchants feel more comfortable doing business with persons of strong religious faith.[20]

And recall from chapter 11 that churchgoing tends to raise living standards in general—to the tune of at least $12,000 in higher family income[21], as well as bigger and better housing thanks to combined paychecks as a result of less divorce.

Piety and Productivity

Chapter 1 mentions the cooperative farms in Israel known as kibbutzim. Not only are members of religious kibbutzim healthier, but they more effectively work as a team and are more productive. Bradley Ruffle of Ben-Gurion University and Richard Sosis of UConn found that the highest levels of cooperation and generosity were among men who engaged in communal prayer, which they did three times daily. And religious kibbutzim outperform secular kibbutzim in agricultural output. For many, this is paradoxical. "Time-consuming and costly religious rituals pose a puzzle for economists committed to rational choice theories of human behavior," write Ruffle and Sosis. It isn't so puzzling to the religiously devout, who believe frequent prayers bring divine assistance. In addition to that, there's greater trust within religious kibbutzim, in which members know that their fellow members are holding themselves accountable to a higher power. This no doubt helps productivity as well. A similar phenomenon occurred during the Middle Ages. Farms worked by Catholic monks were more successful than those worked by serfs, thanks to greater cooperation among the monks.[22]

In a similar vein, the United States in the nineteenth century was home to many secular and religious communes. An anthropologist in the late twentieth century analyzed 200 of them, 112 secular and 88 religious. The secular ones dissolved at a rate up to four times higher than religious ones in any given year. Sheiman attributes that to the greater social cohesiveness religion engenders.[23]

Fostering Faith: A Moral Imperative

With the immense societal benefits, bolstering religious participation and faith-based organizations is of paramount importance. Unfortunately, the opposite is happening. Churchgoing is plummeting and churchlessness skyrocketing. In America's institutions, freedom of worship is being suppressed or eradicated. Vocal prayer and Bible readings in public schools are outlawed. Not even football coaches can lead prayer at games. In school textbooks, references to religious influences in early America are scarce. On college campuses, anti-religion is rampant. At least one professor who wrote about the benefits of religion—as it relates to crime reduction—was fired, as happened to Byron Johnson at Memphis State in the 1980s.[24] (Fortunately, as mentioned in the introduction, these days professors for the most part are free to study the health and societal benefits of religion, but not always.) Christian colleges are in danger of losing their accreditation. The Ten Commandments and other religious imagery on and within government buildings are being removed. There are efforts to remove "under God" from the Pledge of Allegiance, and to end tax exemptions for faith-based nonprofits. When media outlets dole out advice on combatting depression and anxiety, they're usually mum on church and prayer.

In attempting to justify their actions, opponents of religion frequently cite separation of church and state—but it's typically a distortion and misinterpretation thereof. The phrase doesn't even appear in the Constitution—it was coined by Thomas Jefferson afterward. He'd be appalled at efforts today to stifle faith. By separation of church and state, America's Founding Fathers meant prohibiting the establishment of a state-sponsored religion and prohibiting the government from forcing people to accept it. The Founders' intent was to avoid the practice of England at that time, where coercion was institutionalized. They wanted citizens to have free will in choosing their religion. Separation of church and state doesn't mean the government cannot encourage a certain belief system, which is a far cry from coercion into one. The U.S.

government encourages things all the time, such as exercise and eating right. But it doesn't coerce people into doing that. It should adopt the same attitude toward healthy churchgoing. Otherwise, brace yourself for ever-worsening crime, strife, suicide, loneliness, despair, indecency, and material and spiritual impoverishment. As Fagan writes, "To work to reduce the influence of religious belief or practice is to further the disintegration of society."[25]

Chapter 17

REASONS TO BELIEVE

It's a conundrum that public worship and religious affiliation are falling while stark evidence of the physical, medical, emotional, marital, familial, sexual, professional, educational, financial, judicial, communicational, societal, spiritual, eternal, colossal, and monumental benefits of religiosity just keeps piling up.

Holistic health is all the rage these days. Folks travel extra miles to specialty grocers and shell out enormous sums to eat the right foods. They work out for hours on end to tone their muscles and improve their cardiovascular. They spend gargantuan time and money meeting with their therapists. It's all for the sake of striving to live happier, healthier, and longer. But they're missing out on a key wellness booster. Literally thousands of studies, surveys, articles, reviews, and commentaries on the religion-health connection are available for their reading pleasure through a simple Internet query. Have they not come across an article or blog post touting that connection? Was their appetite not whetted to discover more about this fascinating topic? Do they not realize that, as the Harvard researchers deduced, an estimated 40 percent of the rise in suicides and mental illness in recent decades is because of abandonment of devotion to God?[1] Instead of re-embracing faith, people are succumbing to depression, drugs, drink, despair, and death—in droves.

And it isn't just the stark evidence of the wellness benefits of religion that's staring people in the face. It's the stark evidence of religion itself. For some strange reason, many lost souls have been misled into thinking science and religion aren't compatible. Perhaps they could have jumped to that conclusion a hundred or more years ago when science hadn't yet stumbled upon the immensely sophisticated and elaborate engineering not only found in things as tiny as the cell, but as large as the cosmos. Science has progressed so much that all of that is plain to see—not just by biology or astronomy students but by anyone with access to the Internet. Even atheists are admitting as much. A case in point is University of Toronto professor of psychiatry and *Psychology Today* columnist Ralph Lewis:

> "Theism even made a comeback in recent decades, as science revealed the incredible intricacy and complexity of life and the universe. It all seemed too complex, too 'clever' to be unguided. Several enigmas remained seemingly impenetrable. A sophisticated intellectual defense of belief in God usually starts with some version of the argument that the universe must have had a beginning and could not have brought itself into existence: Why is there something rather than nothing? How could something come from nothing? The argument then proceeds to the assertion that the immense complexity of our world could not have arisen spontaneously and unguided."[2]

He makes valiant attempts to explain such new discoveries from an atheistic standpoint, but nevertheless, as evidence of intentional design in nature keeps piling up, such explanations increasingly ring hollow.

Whatever the reasons why religiosity is waning while its personal benefits and intellectual coherence are ever more obvious, at issue right now is you, dear reader. If you've read this far, perhaps you're intrigued by the abundant scholarly research on religiosity and health and are toying with the idea of going to church—or going back to church. Now remember: this book has repeatedly emphasized the importance of doing so for the love of God and not for the love of health. But what if you still haven't brought yourself to fully embrace Him? First, let's go through some of the possibilities along the faith spectrum:

- You're a militant atheist who scorns organized religion.
- You're an atheist who has nothing against organized religion.
- You're agnostic, i.e. you don't know whether there's a God and perhaps don't even care.
- You're the type of agnostic in which you think there's probably a God but that it's impossible to know anything about Him or what He wants out of us, and you're therefore skeptical of any kind of religion.
- You're a deist, in which you believe that once God created the universe, He just let it go on its own without ever subsequently paying attention to it (or to us) or intervening in it.
- You're spiritual but not religious and deem yourself as having no need for organized religion.
- You consider yourself a member of a religion but rarely attend church.
- You usually attend but your heart isn't into it. Perhaps you're only there because of your spouse, your kids, or another reason. You're "extrinsically religious."
- You regularly go to church but your heart is only partially into it; you embrace some or even most of your religion's teachings but not all of them.

One of the above may resemble your situation. If you'd like to believe but aren't quite ready to believe, consider the following discussion. This chapter presents evidence that:

- There is a God.
- He has revealed and continues to reveal Himself.
- He has communicated to us many things about Himself.
- He wants us to not only worship Him but do so in a particular manner.
- He wants us to conduct our lives and treat others according to His teachings.

Space constraints only allow for a brief overview. Take the time to undertake your own more detailed review of the evidence, widely available via books, blogs, articles, videos, podcasts, etc. The deeper you get into it, the more compelling it is. These days it's easier than ever to uncover evidence of the existence of God. It's literally at your fingertips; simply type in "proof of God" or "evidence of God" in a search engine and plentiful web pages and videos will come up. Pre-Internet it was a lot harder to dig up that information, so today we're fortunate in that regard.

Follow the Evidence

Science has progressed so much that it's uncovering things not explainable by science and that point to an intelligent Creator. One is the Big Bang. Prior to the widespread acceptance of this theory, scientists embraced the steady-state theory which holds that the universe always has existed—that it's eternal. They scoffed at the biblical notion that the universe suddenly came into existence out of nothing. But then they learned otherwise. As Robert Jastrow, astrophysicist and founder of NASA's Goddard Institute for Space Studies declared,

> "Now we see how the astronomical evidence supports the biblical view of the origin of the world. All the details differ, but the essential element in the astronomical and biblical accounts of Genesis is the same; the chain of events leading to man commenced suddenly and sharply, at a definite moment in time, in a flash of light and energy."[3]

> "For the scientist who has lived by his faith in the power of reason, the story ends like a bad dream. He has scaled the mountain of ignorance; he is about to conquer the highest peak; as he pulls himself over the final rock, he is greeted by a band of theologians who have been sitting there for centuries."[4]

> "That there are what I or anyone would call supernatural forces at work is now, I think, a scientifically proven fact."[5]

Even more extraordinary is the fine-tuning of the Big Bang and laws of physics. The initial expansion rate of the universe had to be exquisitely exact, calibrated down to 1 in a hundred quadrillion.

Had it been any slower it would have collapsed in on itself. Had it been faster it would have expanded too rapidly for stars to form and life to emerge.[6] The intricate fine-tuning also applies to the magnitudes of the force of gravity, the strong and weak nuclear forces, the electromagnetic force, the speed of light, and several other physical constants or laws of physics.[7]

Imagine a giant round dial with trillions upon trillions of units on it, each less than a nanometer apart. Let's say the force of gravity that sprang up out of the Big Bang could have been any one of those settings. But for planets to form and life to exist, there's just one setting among those trillions of possibilities. Had the dial been turned ever-so-slightly one unit to the right, we wouldn't be here. Same thing if it were one unit to the left. How is it possible the dial was on the precise setting? Just by chance? No. There had to have been an intelligent Creator involved. That's especially the case considering that each of the other physical constants has their own dial and own unique, exact setting. Nearly all astrophysicists agree that all of those physical constants had to have been finely tuned for life to eventually emerge.[8] The odds of that happening on their own were infinitely remote.

There are other instances of fine-tuning in science, such as a phenomenon in chemistry known as resonance levels. Those levels have to be an exact magnitude to get carbon bonding. Sir Fred Hoyle, a prominent cosmologist, went from being an atheist to something of a believer after realizing this couldn't have happened through random chance.[9] He compared the chances of life developing on its own to the chances of a tornado kicking up debris in a junkyard and all of it landing in the form of a perfect Boeing 747 ready for flight.[10]

It's a similar situation vis-à-vis the complex engineering and automated processes that go on inside a cell—vastly more sophisticated than anything humans have ever designed. This couldn't have arisen through random chance. Type in "3D animation cell" or "molecular machines" on the Internet and you'll be amazed at the videos that come up. Tellingly, a YouTube search reveals zero step-by-step animations of how that could have arisen through random chance.

Also compelling is something known as irreducible complexity, a.k.a. purposeful arrangement of parts.[11] Consider the outboard engine of a powerboat. Take away any of the key parts, and it won't work. You can't gradually construct it and expect it will function during points along that assembly process. It won't work until all key parts are in place. It's the same way with cellular-level biological machines such as the bacterial flagellum (see image), which are tiny outboard engines that power bacteria through liquid. The random-chance theory of the origin of life and of biological machines holds that the components came into place gradually over the course of eons. But this doesn't make sense because any partially built machine would have been nonfunctional and useless. A random, impersonal, conscious-less process wouldn't "create" such a thing; it has no future plans in mind. Only a conscious, intelligent Mind with plans for future use of the machine would create it.

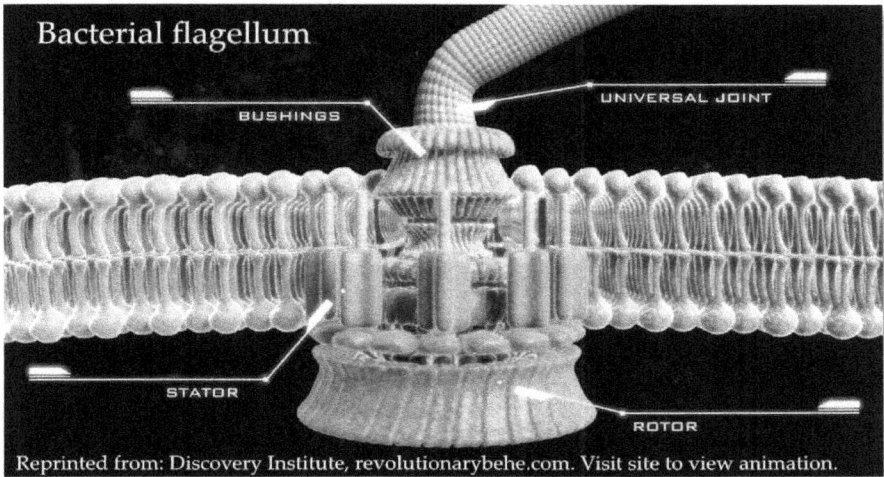

Bacterial flagellum

BUSHINGS

UNIVERSAL JOINT

STATOR

ROTOR

Reprinted from: Discovery Institute, revolutionarybehe.com. Visit site to view animation.

Douglas Axe is a molecular biologist at the Discovery Institute and professor at Biola University. Back in college and grad school he first studied engineering and then switched to biology. He recalls a professor lecturing about an elaborate control circuit in the cell, which turns on and off the production of an amino acid called tryptophan. He sat there dumbfounded, because it was so similar to control systems he had learned about in engineering classes. He knew these biologic control systems couldn't have arisen accidentally by chance. There had to have been an intelligent Creator.[12]

An atheist may still put his fist down and insist there's no intelligent Creator. But in doing that he'd have to admit he's a person of great faith—faith in the power of spontaneous self-assembly. If he can't explain how all of the cellular components randomly assembled themselves into functional machines and processes, then he has to concede that believing that is a leap of faith. To be a bona-fide atheist, he'd also have to explain: how the laws of physics appeared on their own; where quarks came from; how quarks assembled themselves into protons, neutrons, and electrons; how those assembled into atoms; how atoms assembled into molecules; how molecules assembled into DNA and amino acids; how amino acids assembled themselves into proteins; how proteins assembled themselves into cells; how cells assembled into organs; and how organs assembled themselves into living beings. If he can't explain all of that, he has faith in things for which there's no evidence.

Francis Crick, the co-discoverer of DNA, wrote, "An honest man, armed with all the knowledge available to us now, could only state that in some sense, the origin of life appears to be a miracle, so many are the conditions which have had to have been satisfied to get it going."[13] Unfortunately, Crick refused to believe in God. He proposed that the seeds of life came here on a spaceship from some alien civilization.

An origin-of-life theory known as the RNA World hypothesis holds that the evolution of RNA preceded that of DNA and proteins. But according to Scottish chemist Graham Cairns-Smith, forming an RNA involves some 140 steps, and for each step about six reactions have to be avoided. "So, the odds of any starting molecule eventually being converted into RNA is equivalent to throwing a dice and it landing on the number six, 140 times in a row," write Johnjoe McFadden and Jim Al-Khalili in their book *Life on the Edge: The Coming of Age of Quantum Biology*. This is impossible. "Clearly, we cannot rely on pure chance alone," they declare.[14]

But like Crick, they make no mention of evidence of a transcendent Creator. Instead they resort to quantum physics to explain it. But quantum physics involves what seem like little miracles always happening which scientists cannot explain. For example, particles move through solid walls. A single particle can be in multiple places simultaneously. Particles defy the speed of light by having the ability to affect each other instantaneously even though the other particles are billions of light years away. Quantum physics is very supernatural-like. Accepting quantum physics makes it easy to accept there's a supernatural world, and by extension, easy to accept there's a God.

Materialism is the atheistic worldview that only physical matter exists. Quantum physics "destroys materialism completely," argues philosopher and Oxford emeritus professor of divinity Keith Ward. He says materialism has been abandoned by every respectable physicist and philosopher. It's hard for a quantum physicist not to believe in a God, he points out. And the ones who don't believe in God simply do the experiments without bothering with thinking about the why or the how.[15]

God Incarnate

The above are just snippets of the vast literature on evidence for the existence of God. Let's assume you've finally come around to believing in Him. The next logical step is to learn more about Him. What are aspects of His nature, and what does He want out of us? It's those questions the world's religions try to answer. There are five major religions and within those, myriad denominations. They all differ in their conception of God. Which to choose? All too often, people join a religion or denomination based on the one that's most pleasing to them and conforms to their personal preferences. Perhaps it involves an interesting philosophy or trumpets a certain way of life or adopts certain political stances that one finds attractive. But that's not the way to go about selecting a religion. To get to heaven and eternally be in the presence of God, you want to choose the belief system that's most pleasing to *God* and that most conforms to *His* personal preferences, not to our own. How to find that out? Again, follow the evidence.

Let's start by rejecting deism—the belief that God created the universe but doesn't intervene in it and instead just left us to fend for ourselves. This isn't logical. It would imply a cruel God; akin to someone placing various kinds of biting ants into a terrarium and walking away to let them fight. It's rational to conclude that a God who'd go through all the trouble of creating us and the universe wouldn't stop at that and would want to reveal to us things about Himself. He also logically would want to communicate to us a code of conduct. The belief that God is actively involved in our world and in our lives is known as theism, as opposed to deism.

How would He go about communicating with us? By a loud-speaker in the sky? No—through prophets; through speaking directly to certain chosen people (via dreams, visions, locutions, and inspirations) who in turn communicate to the rest of us what He says. Long ago, these messages were written down in the form of a long manuscript called Basic Instructions Before Leaving Earth, better known by its acronym. (Okay so maybe that wasn't what it originally stood for.) How do we know He communicated to us through the Bible and not through other ancient books? Because there's so much historical, archaeological, and circumstantial evidence for the authenticity of the Bible and especially the section of it known as the Gospels.

The Gospels describe the life of Jesus the Christ. He was actually God who came to earth in the form of a man. How do we know Jesus was God? Because he said and implied several times this to be the case. "So what?", you might retort. "You, I, or anyone could claim to be God." But there's a difference. Jesus backed up his words with actions. He performed many miracles throughout the course of his ministry. His greatest miracle was resurrecting himself from the dead. No other person in history has ever done that. That's compelling proof he meant what he said about being God. (To be sure, he didn't begin his ministry proclaiming outright that he was God; had he done that he would have been executed early on, as there was little freedom of speech back then.)

OK, but what about evidence that he performed all of these miracles, and that the rest of the events depicted in the Gospels are true and accurate? The evidence includes:

- Eyewitness accounts in the Gospels themselves. Historians agree that the Gospels were written within decades of Jesus's crucifixion. During that time and afterward, there still were plenty of people alive, including many enemies of Jesus, who would have exposed the Gospels if they were false. No writings have ever been found from around that time period taking issue with events described in the Gospels. Non-Christian texts corroborate many events of Jesus's life, including his miracles. (His detractors attributed the miracles to sorcery.)

- The transformed lives of Jesus's apostles. *The Case for Christ* author Lee Strobel writes, "People will die for their religious beliefs if they sincerely believe they are true, but people won't die for their religious beliefs if they know their beliefs are false."[16] Jesus's apostles and other disciples witnessed his resurrection. Their subsequent actions attested that they were absolutely sure it happened. To defend the truth of that event—and by extension, their conviction Jesus was God—they were willing to endure beatings, torture, starvation, destitution, scorn, ridicule, and for eleven of the twelve apostles, martyrdom. That's impressive testimony that their claims were true. If they secretly knew his resurrection to be false, they would have had no reason or willingness to endure such abuse.

- The Messianic Prophecies of the Old Testament of the Bible. Christ or *Christos* is the Greek translation of the Hebrew word Messiah. Messiah means "Anointed One." Throughout the Old Testament, prophets as directed by God indicated who would be king by anointing that person with holy oil. The Messiah would not be just any king. He would be the ultimate savior or liberator from the (supernatural) forces of evil. Many passages in the Old Testament foretell the coming Messiah. He would be born in Bethlehem (Micah 5:2). He would be despised and rejected (Isaiah 53:3). His hands and feet would be pierced (Psalm 22:16)—despite crucifixion not even having been invented yet. His bones would stay intact (Numbers 9:12); they never broke Jesus's legs at his crucifixion, as was the normal practice. The Old Testament contains dozens of other uncanny predictions of the life of Jesus. How do we know the Old Testament wasn't subsequently changed to make it appear it contained the prophecies? One reason is the discovery of Old Testament sections in the Dead Sea Scrolls, which are dated to two hundred years before the birth of Christ.

These are just a few examples of the overwhelming evidence that Jesus is the Christ and is God. Given this subject's profound importance—at stake is where one will spend eternity—it's incumbent upon any skeptic to undertake his or her own investigation. Never before in history has it been easier to access abundant verification of the authenticity of Jesus and the Gospels. Numerous articles, papers, books, and videos on the subject are available just by typing in a few keywords in a search engine. Good books on the subject include Brant Pitre's *The Case for Jesus* and Lee Strobel's *The Case for Christ*. Books on science-based evidence for God include *New Proofs for the Existence of God* by Robert Spitzer and *The Reality of God* by Steven Hemler.

Mother Church

In the Gospels, Jesus was clear in his directive to build his church. He told the apostle Peter, "You are Peter, and upon this rock I will build my church, and the gates of hell will not prevail against it." (Matthew 16:18) Naturally, his church is still alive and well.

But it seems there are so many churches; which one to choose? Note that Jesus was speaking to Peter when he founded his church. Peter's original name was Simon, but Jesus changed it to Peter which means "rock." Jesus told him he is the rock upon which he will build his church; he made Peter the head of it, which Peter dutifully lived up to during the decades following Jesus's resurrection. When Peter died, the Apostles already had in place a succession plan—not only to replace Peter with a new head of the church but also to replace each of the other Apostles. Those taking their place came to be called bishops, and the leader of them the pope, i.e. the head bishop based in Rome where Peter died. Within a decade or so of Christ's resurrection the followers of Christ started to be called Christians, and decades later they started calling themselves Catholic Christians[17]—catholic means "universal." And that was the way it was for some 1,500 years, during which time there was only one denomination of Jesus's church—apart from minor schisms that died out and a major schism that happened in the year 1054 when Christians in eastern lands decided to not submit to the pope, but they kept everything else mostly the same. Then, by the 1500s unfortunately there was corruption among church leaders in which they strayed from following the teachings of their church. That understandably incensed many Catholics, but rather than working to reform the Mother Church, some decided to break away from it and come up with their own teachings and doctrines. Without a Mother Church, the dissidents started to splinter into many hundreds of denominations, each with their particular teachings that usually contradicted those of other denominations. Now, 500 years later, there are anywhere from a few thousand to more than 35,000 denominations depending on how you count.[18]

If you're looking for a church to join, prayerfully consider joining the Mother Church, the Catholic Church. The Catholic Church is to the Bible what the Supreme Court is to the Constitution. What would happen if we didn't have a supreme authority to interpret, explain, and proclaim the truths of the U.S. Constitution? Then everyone would have their own interpretation/understanding of this 4,400-word document. People would form groups and splinter into factions—maybe even break off to form their own little countries. It would be chaotic. In a similar way, what would happen if there were no supreme authority to interpret, explain, and proclaim the truths of the Bible? Factions galore. It's an ancient, one-million-word document, with many abstruse passages. Just to translate the Bible into English involves the unique interpretation of the translator.

Each reader has his or her own interpretation or understanding of its many teachings and exhortations. This is why beginning from the schism in the 1500s there have grown to be thousands of denominations of Christianity.

Just as God gave us the Bible, it's logical to conclude He would give us a supreme authority to properly interpret it. The Mother Church is still here, just as it has been for the past 2,000 years, serving as the supreme authority on where to go for understanding the teachings of the Bible. An example is when Jesus holds up the bread and wine at the Last Supper. He says "Take, eat; this is my body," and "This is my blood of the covenant." (Matthew 26:26,28) Unlike virtually all other denominations, the Catholic Church takes Jesus's words literally, not figuratively. Earlier Jesus says "Truly, truly, I say to you, unless you eat the flesh of the Son of Man and drink his blood, you have no life in you." Five times in a row. (John 6:53-58) The original Greek word in the Bible for eat is gnaw, or chew—meaning literally to eat. When many of his disciples could not accept this teaching, they walked away. Had Jesus been speaking figuratively, he would have told them so and called them back. But he did not. He was speaking literally. This is why during every Catholic Mass the priest consecrates the bread and wine, called the Eucharist, which the worshipers consume. Based on the aforementioned Bible passages, Catholics believe the Eucharist is the real presence of Christ.

Apart from intellectual evidence of the authenticity of the Gospels and of the Mother Church, there's supernatural evidence. On the Internet, look up English translations of eyewitness newspaper accounts of the Miracle of the Sun that happened in Fatima, Portugal on October 13, 1917. Since May of that year the Blessed Virgin Mary, mother of Jesus, had been appearing to three shepherd children and communicating to them messages from God. She was only visible to the children. So they asked her to give a sign to the tens of thousands of onlookers to prove she truly was appearing to them. She consented, announcing to them a miraculous solar event that would take place around noon October 13. Sure enough, over a crowd of some 70,000 people, on the anticipated day the sun danced in the sky, making various movements, colors, and shapes. Science cannot explain it, and no one has debunked it. The event proved the Blessed Mother actually had been appearing to the children. So how does this prove the authenticity of the Catholic Church? Because everything she told the children was consistent with the teachings of the Church. This includes the reality of not only hell but of purgatory, the need to carry out penances and make sacrifices to save one's soul and the souls of others, the importance of receiving the Eucharist, and the importance of praying the Rosary frequently. In addition to Fatima, there have been many, many authenticated appearances of the Blessed Virgin Mary around the world, all with a consistent message.

God has a plan for us. It's logical to conclude that the God who created us would reveal to us in detail not only things about His nature but also what He expects of us and how He wants us to live our lives. That's all found in the Bible. And the historical evidence that Jesus Christ rose from the dead is compelling evidence that the Bible is true—not necessarily each story and parable in it, but rather the messages of the Bible. Because the Bible can be difficult to understand and interpret, it also is logical to conclude that our God would give us a supreme authority, guided by the Holy Spirit, to properly interpret the Bible and to carry out the directives set forth by its central figure, Jesus Christ. That supreme authority is the 2,000-year-old Catholic Church. (A good book on this subject is Scott Hahn's *Rome Sweet Home*.)

New Catholic Blood

One reason so many have fallen away from the faith of their youth is they never heard any proofs of the existence of God, especially science-related proofs. They never were taught historical evidence of the authenticity of the Gospels and of Jesus's resurrection. Among Catholics or former Catholics, they never were presented with biblical evidence of the foundations of their faith. These themes fall under the rubric known as apologetics. To be sure, this has nothing to do with apologizing for anything. Apologetics means explaining and defending the faith with logical reasoning and presentation of evidence. The word comes from the Greek *apologia*, which means "speaking in defense," as in presenting the defense in legal proceedings. It only was around the late 16th century (possibly based on a Shakespeare play) when the word started morphing into the "I'm sorry" meaning.

For some inexplicable reason, apologetics is commonly given short shrift by religious leaders. Upon hearing a sermon or lecture about a Gospel passage or other aspect of the faith, no doubt a key question in the minds of many is, "That's all well and good but how do I know it's true?" Priests, bishops, ministers, and religious educators rarely seem to cater to the doubters. This no doubt is why droves of people leave their churches. Catholic schools and religious education programs sometimes teach apologetics, but it typically is an apologetics more geared toward 50 to 100 years ago when the main debate in America was Catholicism versus Protestantism rather than today when the main debate is between Christianity and atheism/agnosticism or New Ageism. As mentioned in chapter 9, another dereliction of duty by Catholic clergy and educators is in the area of sexual ethics, even though this subject is so prominent in Church doctrines. With a lack of apologetics and lack of firm guidance on sexual ethics, it's no wonder that so many people have left the Church, so few save sex until marriage, and so many are addicted to porn.

But these days you need not rely on your local priest or religion teacher to learn about God and his Church (but you still need a Catholic priest in order to consume Christ's body and blood). You can learn about it on your own thanks to the Internet, books, videos, podcasts, and other such media. Uninspiring sermons? Keep going to Mass and receiving the Holy Eucharist, and afterward listen to a sermon online from an inspiring and charismatic priest.

Another bright spot is that the younger generation of Catholic priests generally are much more orthodox and "on fire for the faith" than older generations of priests, portending well for the future of the Church. They have a reputation for being morally upright, unlike some in the older generation who had little fear of God (and possibly little belief in Him) and consequently slid into sin and scandal, ushering in the sexual abuse crisis. The vast majority of that happened in the 1960s, 1970s, and 1980s when confusion and laxity reigned following the Second Vatican Council. Today, with many of those excesses recognized and reigned in, the Church is in much better shape.

Psychotherapy for Free

The spiritual benefits of the Catholic Church are legion. To quote Father Michael Gaitley, it's the "surest, easiest, shortest, and most perfect means" to get to heaven. That's especially so when it's through a devotion to the Blessed Virgin Mary.[19] But apart from improving your spiritual health for the hereafter, the Catholic Church offers some of the best tools available for boosting emotional health for the here and now. It's no coincidence that, as discussed in chapter 10, there were no suicides among the 7,000 Catholics in the Nurses' Health Study who said they attend Mass more than once a week. If weekly churchgoing has so many wellness benefits, imagine what daily churchgoing can do (and most Catholic churches offer daily Mass).

Plus there's confession. It's like a mini-psychotherapy session for free—with spiritual healing to boot. Take it from the eminent psychiatrist and psychoanalyst Carl Jung: "Confession sometimes has a truly redeeming effect. The tremendous feeling of relief which usually follows a confession can be ascribed to the readmission of the lost sheep into the human community. His moral isolation and seclusion, which were so difficult to bear, cease. Herein lies the chief psychological value of confession."[20]

It's thanks in part to self-forgiveness and knowledge that one is forgiven by God that confession is so beneficial to emotional health. As reported by Robert Todd Wise in his Ph.D. dissertation on the healing power of confession, penitents speak of "a sense of relief, of healing, of empowerment that an obstacle had been overcome…

Forgiveness was accepted as a gift of Grace." He adds, "They underwent feelings of empowerment, elation, cleanness, renewal, joy, and peace. Some penitents experienced these positive feelings for an extended period following a confession. Penitents described the benefits received in the confessional as cathartic and as healing, i.e. healing of a low sense of self-worth."[21]

Scholars have found in humans a "compulsion to confession," and that when it's carried out, it's "profoundly healing physically, psychologically, and spiritually," writes psychologist Aaron Murray-Swank—even when it's not in the context of a Catholic confession booth or involving a third party. He points to a study that examined the effects of disclosing personal thoughts and feelings. Though there could be some immediate distress, over time it turned out that participants enjoyed better mood, less psychological distress, less illness, and even improved immune functioning.[22]

Another tool for enhancing spiritual and emotional well-being is what's known as Eucharistic Adoration, in which a consecrated communion host—called the Eucharist, which Catholics believe is the real body and blood of Christ—is prominently displayed in an elegant holder (known as a monstrance) in a small chapel inside a Catholic church. Anyone—Catholic or not—can sit in solitude before it for as long as he or she wishes, to pray, read, or just get away from the hustle and bustle of daily life. People testify that doing this is the most peaceful, satisfying hour of their week. Such chapels often are open to the public twenty-four hours a day, several days a week. As one chaplain observed, many have spoken of being touched by God at Eucharistic Adoration, "either feeling God's love in a particular way that brings them to tears, or a lifting of a burden, or they sense God's presence in a way that they feel a healing."[23]

Giving Back to God

Let's say you'd like to start going to church but you're holding off because you don't think your faith is strong enough yet to be intrinsically religious. Don't delay—go there anyway. Repeated exposure to religious practice and frequent interaction with other churchgoers will help you develop spiritually. Typically, a convergence of factors gets a person on fire for the faith, prompting the Holy Spirit to take hold. In addition to apologetics, such factors may include:

- a dynamic or inspiring pastor or other church leader.
- inspirational friends and others you meet at church who are fervent for the Lord.
- reading the Bible and especially the Gospels.
- watching and reading on the Internet the abundant personal testimonies of how lives were transformed by embracing God.
- viewing and perusing on the Internet and in books the many amazing accounts of near-death experiences.
- going on a retreat or other faith-based organized event.
- visiting a religious pilgrimage site.
- attending a Bible-focused or other spirituality group that meets regularly.
- joining a church-sponsored men's or women's group.
- doing charity work and seeing the face of Jesus in the poor.
- reading spiritual books and taking in other faith-based media.
- saying prayers that get answered.
- a mystical experience, where you're convinced you had a supernatural encounter (but this is rare).
- being convinced of mystical experiences of others, as described in books, blogs, video testimonies, and/or by someone you know.
- becoming convinced of miraculous phenomena such as medically unexplainable physical healings or other extraordinary events not attributable to science or coincidence.

Once at church, initially or later on you may feel like you're not getting anything out of it. That's what prompts a lot of people to stop going. But they have it backward. Church isn't supposed to be what *you* get out of it. It's supposed to be what *God* gets out of it. It's about worshiping *Him*. All God asks is that you take one simple hour out of your 168-hour week to pay Him homage. Even if you feel bored or that you're not learning anything or the priest or minister is unremarkable or the music is dull or you're not getting any tingly sensations, that doesn't matter. God wants to see you making the very modest effort of sitting for an hour in one of His houses of worship, just to acknowledge Him; to give a little something back to Him considering the abundance He has given you. It's not very much to ask. You may not feel them, but you're getting graces galore. You'll get to see their real value after you step into the next world.

Mental Eclipses Physical

The next world is what this short life is all about. Our present life is a testing ground to demonstrate our love for God and for fellow human beings in order to be admitted into His heavenly kingdom when our time comes. This evokes the question, what's more important: good physical health, or good mental health? It's mental health. From an eternal salvation standpoint, it matters not how long you live or what diseases you get, but what you did to please God while you were alive. In the words of fifteenth-century monk Thomas à Kempis, "It is vanity to wish for long life and to care little about a well-spent life."[24] Longevity is not necessarily an advantage for spiritual health. If someone turns against God and His teachings yet lives a long life, it means more years of displeasing God. Meanwhile a shorter life could eliminate the possibility of someone eventually choosing to rebel against Him. On the other hand, for someone else a long life could be a good thing spiritually: more years to engage in church, prayer, penance, and good works. That's particularly advantageous if you only started embracing God later in life.

Physical diseases and disabilities aren't sins; they could be blessings in disguise if they shake the person into caring more about God and neighbor. On the mental side, things are more problematic. Depression and anxiety certainly aren't sins. But despair, rage, unforgiveness, alcohol abuse, drug abuse, divorce (in most cases, for at least one party), suicide, and delinquency are. Yes, even despair is considered a sin, at least in the Catholic tradition, because it implies giving up hope in the mercy and goodness of God. So it's important to embrace church if only to help avoid those above-named transgressions—and improve your mental health to boot.

No Guarantees

Churchgoing will increase the likelihood of you becoming happier and healthier. But it won't guarantee it. You still could get depressed. You still could get chronically ill. You still could come to an end of your earthly life sooner rather than later.

In a similar vein, Jesus never guaranteed health and happiness to his followers. He declared, "Enter by the narrow gate...for the gate is narrow and the way is hard that leads to life, and those who find it are few." (Matthew 7:13-14) St. Paul wrote in the New Testament, "As servants of God we commend ourselves in every way: through great endurance, in afflictions, hardships, calamities..." (2 Corinthians 6:4).

Huh? That's quite a paradox. How can going to church result in health and happiness when Jesus seems to say just the opposite will happen to you? Because you can suffer yet still be of sound mind and body. It's a different kind of suffering. Instead of the early-onset heart disease, weak immune system, depression, alcoholism, drug abuse, marital discord, and suicidal thoughts that you may endure as an atheist or nominal Christian, as a committed Christian the "suffering" could include: getting up earlier on Sunday mornings than you're accustomed to; taking time out of each day to pray; volunteering at a soup kitchen; donating real money to charity; avoiding unnecessary work or shopping on Sundays; holding your tongue when you feel like lashing out; turning down that third drink; reading the spiritual book instead of the popular bestseller; dressing modestly instead of the popular fashion; buying a mild-mannered Honda rather than that flashy BMW; shunning websites with pictures of scantily clad figures; and/or drastically scaling back your time spent on social media.

There are other, more difficult kinds of suffering. It could include being ridiculed or ostracized for holding certain beliefs while those around you cling to the ways of the world. It may involve

not getting a job you applied for, or losing your job, or getting rep-
rimanded, or losing a big client because of your beliefs, or getting
censored, fined, sued, deplatformed, or canceled. You could risk
the loss of friendships or the alienation of family members. In a
worst-case scenario you'd be willing to be imprisoned, tortured,
and die for Jesus.

Jesus told his disciples, "If any man would come after me, let
him deny himself and take up his cross and follow me." (Matthew
16:24) That means, at the cost of our personal lives, we should be
ready and willing to do for him what he did for us when he picked
up that cross and dragged it up to the place where he endured the
ultimate sacrifice.

The Beatitudes in the Bible are where Jesus says blessed are the
poor in spirit, blessed are the mournful, blessed are the meek, blessed are those who hunger and thirst for righteousness, blessed are
the merciful, blessed are the clean of heart, blessed are the peace-
makers, blessed are those who are persecuted for righteousness'
sake, and blessed are those who are reviled and spoken against
falsely for Jesus's sake. "Blessed" is often translated as "happy."
The paradox referred to above is explained by knowing that this is
not an ephemeral, superficial happiness that Jesus is talking about.
It's a real and lasting happiness that only can be satisfied by a close
relationship with him. He says at the end of the Beatitudes, "Re-
joice and be glad, because great is your reward in heaven." This
very much sounds like health and happiness both in this life, and
in the next.

For more on the religion-health relationship, apologetics,
and other intriguing topics, visit seventimes70.com.

References

Introduction

1. Robert A. Hummer, Richard G. Rogers, Charles B. Nam, and Christopher G. Ellison, "Religious Involvement and U.S. Adult Mortality," *Demography,* May 1999, Vol. 36, No. 2, 273-285.

2. Jeff Levin, *God, Faith, and Health: Exploring the Spirituality-Healing Connection,* John Wiley & Sons, 2001, p. 31.

3. Byron R. Johnson, Ralph Brett, and Derek Webb, *Objective Hope: Assessing the Effectiveness of Faith-Based Organizations,* Center for Research on Religion and Urban Civil Society, University of Pennsylvania, 2002.

4. Ibid.

5. Jonathan Gruber, "Religious Market Structure, Religious Participation, and Outcomes: Is Religion Good for You?," National Bureau of Economic Research working paper 11377, May 2005.

6. Megan Brenan, "Americans' Mental Health Ratings Sink to New Low," Gallup news story, Dec. 7, 2020, https://news.gallup.com/poll/327311/americans-mental-health-ratings-sink-new-low.aspx.

7. Shuli Brammli-Greenberg, Jacob Glazer, and Ephraim Shapiro, "The Inverse U-Shaped Religion-Health Connection Among Israeli Jews," *Journal of Religion and Health,* Feb. 2018, Vol. 57, No. 2, pp. 738-750.

8. For a summary of a systematic review of the research, see Harold Koenig, "Religion, Spirituality, and Health: The Research and Clinical Implications," *ISRN Psychiatry,* Dec. 2012, Article ID 278730.

9. Kashmira Gander, "'Deaths of Despair': U.S. Life Expectancy Has Been Falling Since 2014, With Biggest Impacts in Rust Belt and Ohio Valley," *Newsweek,* Nov. 26, 2019.

10. Tyler VanderWeele, Shanshan Li, and Ichiro Kawachi, reply to letter to the editor concerning "Religious Service Attendance and Suicide Rates," *JAMA Psychiatry,* Feb. 2017, Vol. 74, Issue 2. Also: Tyler VanderWeele, e-mail communication with author, May 5, 2021.

11. Based on comments to author from Tyler VanderWeele and Jeff Levin.

12. Tyler J. VanderWeele, "Religion and Health: A Synthesis," In: Peteet, J.R. and Balboni, M.J. (Eds.), *Spirituality and Religion within the Culture of Medicine: From Evidence to Practice,* Oxford University Press, 2017.

13. Joel James Shuman and Keith G. Meador, *Heal Thyself: Spirituality, Medicine, and the Distortion of Christianity,* Oxford University Press, 2003, p. 21.

14. Andrew Newberg, "The Spiritual Brain: Science and Religious Experience," The Great Courses series, lecture 10, July 2013.

15. Paul Pavao, "2 Clement: The Earliest Christian Sermon," Christian History for Everyman, christian-history.org. https://www.christian-history.org/2-clement.html.

16. Yoichi Chida, Andrew Steptoe, and Linda H. Powell, "Religiosity/Spirituality and Mortality: A Systematic Quantitative Review," *Psychotherapy and Psychosomatics,* Jan. 2009, Vol. 78, Issue 78, pp. 81-90.

17. Tyler VanderWeele, telephone interview with author, March 1, 2021.

Chapter 1: Bolster Your Bodily Health

1. Harold G. Koenig, *Is Religion Good for Your Health? The Effects of Religion on Physical and Mental Health*, The Haworth Pastoral Press, 1997, p. 80.
2. Vanessa Dirwai, "God Has Helped Me Get My Health Back - IBS, EDS, Joint PAIN - Health Journey," YouTube, Nov. 3, 2019, https://youtu.be/CNn04XhASpA.
3. Harold G. Koenig, Linda K. George, Harvey J. Cohen, Judith C. Hays, David B. Larson, and Dan G. Blazer, "The Relationship Between Religious Activities and Cigarette Smoking in Older Adults," *The Journals of Gerontology: Series A*, Nov. 1998, Vol. 53A, Issue 6, pp. M426-M434.
4. Joanna Tully, Russell M. Viner, Pietro G. Coen, James M. Stuart, Maria Zambon, Catherine Peckham, Clare Booth, Nigel Klein, Ed Kaczmarski, and Robert Booy, "Risk and Protective Factors for Meningococcal Disease in Adolescents: Matched Cohort Study," Feb. 2006, *The BMJ*, Vol. 332, Issue 7539, pp. 445-450.
5. Harold G. Koenig and David B. Larson, "Use of Hospital Services, Religious Attendance, and Religious Affiliation," *Southern Medical Journal*, Oct. 1998, Vol. 91, No. 9, pp. 925-932.
6. Spirituality in Patient Care video series, part 1. Center for Spirituality, Theology and Health, Duke University.
7. "Dr. Harold Koenig Faith and Health," YouTube video, Healthy Human Revolution channel, Jan. 28, 2019, https://www.youtube.com/watch?v=asS4gnu-aII.
8. Franco Bonaguidi, Claudio Michelassi, Franco Filipponi, and Daniele Rova, "Religiosity Associated with Prolonged Survival in Liver Transplant Recipients," *Liver Transplantation*, 2010, Vol. 16, pp. 1158-1163.
9. William J. Strawbridge, Sarah J. Shema, Richard D. Cohen, and George A Kaplan, "Religious Attendance Increases Survival by Improving and Maintaining Good Health Behaviors, Mental Health, and Social Relationships," *Annals of Behavioral Medicine*, Feb. 2001, Vol. 23, No. 1, pp. 68-74.
10. Ellen L. Idler and Stanislav V. Kasl, "Religion Among Disabled and Nondisabled Persons II: Attendance at Religious Services as a Predictor of the Course of Disability," *Journal of Gerontology Series B*, Dec. 1997, Vol. 52B, No. 6, pp. S306-S316.
11. Harold G. Koenig, Ellen L. Idler, Stanislav Kasl, Judith C. Hays, Linda K. George, Marc Musick, David B. Larson, Terence Collins, and Herbert Benson, "Religion, Spirituality, and Medicine: A Rebuttal to Skeptics," Feb. 1999, *The International Journal of Psychiatry in Medicine*, Vol. 29, No. 2, pp. 123-131.
12. Harold Koenig, telephone interview with author, March 16, 2021.
13. Shanshan Li, Meir J. Stampfer, David R. Williams, and Tyler J. VanderWeele, "Association of Religious Service Attendance With Mortality Among Women," *JAMA Internal Medicine*, June 2016, Vol. 176, No. 6, pp. 777-785; Carina Storrs, "Going to Church Could Help You Live Longer, Study Says," CNN, May 16, 2016.
14. Lynda H. Powell, Leila Shahabi, and Carl E. Thoresen, "Religion and Spirituality: Linkages to Physical Health," *American Psychologist*, Jan. 2003.
15. Claudia Kalb, "Faith & Healing," *Newsweek*, Nov. 9, 2003, https://www.newsweek.com/faith-healing-133365.
16. Yoichi Chida, Andrew Steptoe, and Linda H. Powell, "Religiosity/Spirituality and Mortality: A Systematic Quantitative Review," *Psychotherapy and Psychosomatics*, Jan. 2009, Vol. 78, Issue 78, pp. 81-90.
17. Michael E. McCullough, William T. Hoyt, David B. Larson, Harold G. Koenig, and Carl Thoresen, "Religious Involvement and Mortality: A Meta-Analytic

Review," *Health Psychology*, 2000, Vol. 19, No. 3.

18. J.D. Kark, G. Shemi, Y. Friedlander, O. Martin, O. Manor, and S.H. Blondheim, "Does Religious Observance Promote Health? Mortality in Secular vs. Religious Kibbutzim in Israel," *American Journal of Public Health*, Mar. 1996, Vol. 86, No. 3, pp. 341-346.

19. Tyler J. VanderWeele, "Religion and Health: A Synthesis," In: Peteet, J.R. and Balboni, M.J. (Eds.), *Spirituality and Religion within the Culture of Medicine: From Evidence to Practice*, Oxford University Press, 2017.

20. Robert A. Hummer, Richard G. Rogers, Charles B. Nam, and Christopher G. Ellison, "Religious Involvement and U.S. Adult Mortality," *Demography*, May 1999, Vol. 36, No. 2, pp. 273-285.

21. Robert Hummer, "Religious Involvement and U.S. Adult Mortality Risk" PowerPoint presentation, https://www.cdc.gov/nchs/ppt/nchs2010/37_hummer.pdf.

22. Ibid.

23. Ryan Jaslow, "Bachelor's Degree Boosts Health, CDC Report Suggests," CBS News, May 16, 2012, https://www.cbsnews.com/news/bachelors-degree-boosts-health-cdc-report-suggests/.

24. Ibid.

25. Howard S. Friedman and Leslie R. Martin, *The Longevity Project*, Penguin Group, 2012, p. 155-156.

26. Laura E. Wallace, Rebecca Anthony, Christian M. End, and Baldwin M. Way, "Does Religion Stave Off the Grave? Religious Affiliation in One's Obituary and Longevity," *Social Psychological and Personality Science*, June 2018, Vol. 10, Issue 5, pp. 662-670.

27. Daniel E. Hall, "Religious Attendance: More Cost-Effective Than Lipitor?," *Journal of the American Board of Family Medicine*, March-April 2006, Vol. 19, No. 2, pp. 103-109.

28. Duck-chul Lee, Angelique G. Brellenthin, Paul D. Thompson, Xuemei Sui, I-Min Lee, and Carl J. Laviee, "Running as a Key Lifestyle Medicine for Longevity," *Progress in Cardiovascular Diseases*, July-Aug. 2017, Vol. 60, Issue 1, pp. 45-55.

29. Harold G. Koenig, Linda K. George, Judith C. Hays, David B. Larson, Harvey J. Cohen, and Dan G. Blazer, "The Relationship Between Religious Activities and Blood Pressure in Older Adults," *The International Journal of Psychiatry in Medicine*, June 1998, Vol. 28, Issue 2, pp. 189-213.

30. David B. Larson, Harold G. Koenig, Berton H. Kaplan, Raymond S. Greenberg, Everett Logue, Herman A. Tyroler, and Raymond F. Greenberg, "The Impact of Religion on Men's Blood Pressure," *Journal of Religion and Health*, Winter 1989, Vol. 28, No. 4, pp. 265-278.

31. Marino A. Bruce, David Martins, Kenrik Duru, Bettina M. Beech, Mario Sims, Nina Harawa, Roberto Vargas, Dulcie Kermah, Susanne B. Nicholas, Arleen Brown, and Keith C. Norris, "Church Attendance, Allostatic Load and Mortality in Middle Aged Adults," *PLoS ONE*, May 2017, Vol. 12, Issue 5.

32. Byron R. Johnson, Ralph Brett, and Derek Webb, *Objective Hope: Assessing the Effectiveness of Faith-Based Organizations*, Center for Research on Religion and Urban Civil Society, University of Pennsylvania, 2002.

33. Harold Koenig, "Religion, Spirituality, and Health: The Research and Clinical Implications," *ISRN Psychiatry*, Dec. 2012, Article ID 278730.

34. Ellen L. Idler and Stanislav V. Kasl, "Religion Among Disabled and Nondis-

abled Persons II: Attendance at Religious Services as a Predictor of the Course of Disability," *Journal of Gerontology Series B*, Dec. 1997, Vol. 52B, No. 6, pp. S306-S316.
35. Doug Oman and Dwayne Reed, "Religion and Mortality Among the Community-Dwelling Elderly," *American Journal of Public Health*, 1998, Vol. 88, pp. 1469-1475.
36. William J. Strawbridge, Richard D. Cohen, Sarah J. Shema, and George A. Kaplan, "Frequent Attendance at Religious Services and Mortality Over 28 Years," *American Journal of Public Health*, July 1997, Vol. 87, No. 6.
37. Terrence D. Hill, Jacqueline L. Angel, Christopher G. Ellison, and Ronald J. Angel, "Religious Attendance and Mortality: An 8-Year Follow-Up of Older Mexican Americans," *The Journals of Gerontology: Series B*, Vol. 60, Issue 2, pp. S102-S109.
38. Mira Hidajat, Zachary Zimmer, Yasuhiko Saito, and Hui-Sheng Lin, "Religious Activity, Life Expectancy, and Disability-Free Life Expectancy in Taiwan," *European Journal of Ageing*, 2013, Vol. 10, pp. 229-236.
39. Wei Zhang, "Religious Participation and Mortality Risk Among the Oldest Old in China," *The Journals of Gerontology: Series B*, Sept. 2008, Vol. 63, Issue 5.
40. Jeffrey W. Dwyer, Leslie L. Clarke, and Michael K. Miller, "The Effect of Religious Concentration and Affiliation on County Cancer Mortality Rates," *Journal of Health and Social Behavior*, Vol. 31, No. 2, June 1990.
41. Eric C. Shattuck and Michael P Muehlenbein, "Religiosity/Spirituality and Physiological Markers of Health," *Journal of Religion and Health*, April 2020, Vol. 59, Issue 3.
42. Rachael Link, "8 Health Benefits of Fasting, Backed by Science," *Healthline*, July 30, 2018, https://www.healthline.com/nutrition/fasting-benefits.
43. Steven Salzberg, "Can Intermittent Fasting Reset Your Immune System?," *Forbes*, Jan 6, 2020.
44. "11 Health Benefits of Cold Showers, *Insight State*, March 10, 2019, https://www.insightstate.com/health/cold-showers/.
45. Diana M. Zuckerman, Stanislav V. Kasl, and Adrian M. Ostfeld, "Psychosocial Predictors of Mortality Among the Elderly Poor," *American Journal of Epidemiology*, 1984, Vol. 119, Issue 3, pp. 410-423.
46. Linda H. Powell, Leila Shahabi, and Carl E. Thoresen, "Religion and Spirituality: Linkages to Physical Health," *American Psychologist*, Jan. 2003, Vol. 58, No 1.
47. Byron R. Johnson, Ralph Brett, and Derek Webb, *Objective Hope: Assessing the Effectiveness of Faith-Based Organizations*, Center for Research on Religion and Urban Civil Society, University of Pennsylvania, 2002.

Chapter 2: The Psycho-Social Affects the Physical

1. Jared Diamond, *The World Until Yesterday: What Can We Learn from Traditional Societies?*, Viking Adult, 2012, p. 273.
2. Clay Stanton, answer to the Quora question, "How has being a follower of Christ changed your life?," Quora.com, Jan. 24, 2018, https://www.quora.com/How-has-being-a-follower-of-Christ-changed-your-life?share=1.
3. Chaeyoon Lim and Robert D. Putnam, "Religion, Social Networks, and Life Satisfaction," *American Sociological Review*, Dec. 2010, Vol. 75, No. 6, pp. 914-933.
4. Thomas E. Oxman, Daniel H. Freeman Jr., and Eric D. Manheimer, "Lack of Social Participation or Religious Strength and Comfort as Risk Factors for Death After Cardiac Surgery in the Elderly," *Psychosomatic Medicine*, Jan.-Feb. 1995, Vol. 57, Issue 1, pp. 5-15. Also: "Harold Koenig | Spirituality into Clinical Practice," YouTube

video, Feb. 4, 2020, https://www.youtube.com/watch?v=hb0nEaeqAjU&t=1951s.

5. Eran Shor and David J. Roelfs, "The Longevity Effects of Religious and Nonreligious Participation: A Meta-Analysis and Meta-Regression," *Journal for the Scientific Study of Religion*," 2013, Vol. 52, No. 1, pp. 120-145.

6. Simone Croezen, Mauricio Avendano, Alex Burdorf, and Frank J. van Lenthe, "Social Participation and Depression in Old Age: A Fixed-Effects Analysis in 10 European Countries," *American Journal of Epidemiology*, May 2015, Vol. 182, No. 2.

7. Jeff Levin, *God, Faith, and Health: Exploring the Spirituality-Healing Connection*, John Wiley & Sons, 2001, p. 134.

8. Patricia A. Boyle, Lisa L. Barnes, Aron S. Buchman, and David A. Bennett, "Purpose in Life is Associated with Mortality Among Community-Dwelling Older Persons," *Psychosomatic Medicine*, June 2009, Vol. 71, Issue 5, p. 574-579.

9. Patricia A. Boyle, Aron S. Buchman, Lisa L. Barnes, and David A. Bennett, "Effect of a Purpose in Life on Risk of Incident Alzheimer Disease and Mild Cognitive Impairment in Community-Dwelling Older Persons," *Archives of General Psychiatry*, March 2010, Vol. 67, No. 3, pp. 304-310.

10. Neal Krause, "Church-Based Social Support and Health in Old Age: Exploring Variations by Race," *The Journals of Gerontology, Series B: Psychological Sciences and Social Sciences*, Dec. 2002, Vol. 57B, Issue 6, pp. S332-S347.

11. Andrew Newberg, "The Spiritual Brain: Science and Religious Experience," The Great Courses series, lecture 1, July 2013.

12. Jessica Tartaro, Linda Luecken, and Heather Gunn, "Exploring Heart and Soul: Effects of Religiosity/Spirituality and Gender on Blood Pressure and Cortisol Stress Responses," *Journal of Health Psychology*," Vol 10, No. 6, 2005. Also: Talya Steinberg and Ron Breazeale, "Thoughts, Neurotransmitters, Body-Mind Connection," *Psychology Today*, July 12, 2012, https://www.psychologytoday.com/us/blog/in-the-face-adversity/201207/thoughts-neurotransmitters-body-mind-connection. Also: Jeff Levin, *God, Faith, and Health: Exploring the Spirituality-Healing Connection*, John Wiley & Sons, 2001, p. 86.

13. Charles Zeiders, "The Psychophysiology of The Jesus Prayer," drzeiders.com, July 11, 2013, https://drzeiders.com/religion-and-spirituality/the-psychophysiology-of-the-jesus-prayer.

14. "Anger, Hostility and Depressive Symptoms Linked to High C-reactive Protein Levels," *Science Daily*, Sept. 23, 2004, https://www.sciencedaily.com/releases/2004/09/040922070643.htm.

15. Brett Smith, "Good Emotions Lower Inflammation, Study Says," *RedOrbit*, Feb. 4, 2015, https://www.redorbit.com/news/health/1113327832/good-emotions-lower-inflammation-study-says-020415/.

16. David Hanscom, "10 Ways to Lower Cytokines (Thrive) and Survive COVID-19," *Psychology Today*, May 27, 2020, https://www.psychologytoday.com/us/blog/anxiety-another-name-pain/202005/10-ways-lower-cytokines-thrive-and-survive-covid-19.

17. Jeff Levin, *God, Faith, and Health: Exploring the Spirituality-Healing Connection*, John Wiley & Sons, 2001, pp. 80-81. Also Michael E. McCullough, "Prayer and Health: Conceptual Issues, Research Review, and Research Agenda," Journal of Psychology and Theology, Vol. 23, pp 15-29.

18. Jeff Levin, *God, Faith, and Health: Exploring the Spirituality-Healing Connection*, John Wiley & Sons, 2001, pp. 89-90.

19. Spirituality in Patient Care video series, part 2. Center for Spirituality, Theology and Health, Duke University.

20. Joseph K. Neumann and David S. Chi, "Relationship of Church Giving to Immunological and Txpa Stress Response," *Journal of Psychology and Theology*, March 1, 1999, Vol. 27, Issue 1, pp. 43-51.

21. Ryan King, "My Testimony | How Jesus Saved Me From Alcohol, Cigarettes, Anger, Depression, and Hell!," YouTube, May 23, 2020, https://youtu.be/WE7efR-J4lG4.

22. Tyler J. VanderWeele, "Religion and Health: A Synthesis," In: Peteet, J.R. and Balboni, M.J. (Eds.), *Spirituality and Religion within the Culture of Medicine: From Evidence to Practice*, Oxford University Press, 2017.

23. "Are Religious Older Adults Less Susceptible to Infection?", *Crossroads*, newsletter of the Center for Spirituality, Theology and Health, Duke University, Vol. 10, Issue 3, Sept 2020.

24. Luskin, Frederic, *Forgive for Good: A Proven Prescription for Health and Happiness*, HarperCollins, 2002, pp. xv, 79, 87.

25. Patricia P. Chang, Daniel E. Ford, Lucy A. Meoni, Nae-Yuh Wang, and Michael J. Klag, "Anger in Young Men and Subsequent Premature Cardiovascular Disease: The Precursors Study," *Archives of Internal Medicine*, 2002, Vol. 162, Issue 8, pp. 901-906.

26. Janice E. Williams, Catherine C. Paton, Ilene C. Siegler, Marsha L. Eigenbrodt, F. Javier Nieto, and Herman A. Tyroler, "Anger Proneness Predicts Coronary Heart Disease Risk: Prospective Analysis From the Atherosclerosis Risk In Communities (ARIC) Study," *Circulation*, May 2000, Vol. 101, pp. 2034-2039.

27. Daniel Escher, "How Does Religion Promote Forgiveness? Linking Beliefs, Orientations, and Practices," *Journal for the Scientific Study of Religion*, March 2013, Vol. 52, No. 1, pp. 100-119.

28. Nathaniel M. Lambert, Frank D. Fincham, Tyler F. Stillman, Steven M. Graham, and Steven R.H. Beach, "Motivating Change in Relationships: Can Prayer Increase Forgiveness?," *Psychological Science*, Jan. 2010, Vol. 21, No. 1.

29. Neal Krause and Christopher G. Ellison. "Forgiveness by God, Forgiveness of Others, and Psychological Well-Being in Late Life," *Journal for the Scientific Study of Religion*, March 2003, Vol. 42, No. 1, pp. 77-93.

30. "Benefits of Forgiveness on Health," Mudahamatan blog, https://mudahamatan.home.blog/2019/06/19/benefits-of-forgiveness-on-health/.

31. Neal Krause and Christopher G. Ellison. "Forgiveness by God, Forgiveness of Others, and Psychological Well-Being in Late Life," *Journal for the Scientific Study of Religion*, March 2003, Vol. 42, Issue 1, pp. 77-93.

32. Tyler J. VanderWeele, "Religion and Health: A Synthesis," In: Peteet, J.R. and Balboni, M.J. (Eds.), *Spirituality and Religion within the Culture of Medicine: From Evidence to Practice*. New York, NY: Oxford University Press, 2017.

33. Ibid.

34. "Federal Agencies Partner for Military and Veteran Pain Management Research," National Institutes of Health press release, Sept. 20, 2017.

35. Christina Rush, Kaitlyn Vagnini, and Amy Wachholtz, "Spirituality/Religion and Pain," in *Handbook of Spirituality, Religion, and Mental Health*, second edition, David H. Rosmarin and Harold G. Koenig (Eds.), Academic Press, an imprint of Elsevier, 2020.

36. Haleh Tajadini, Nasser Zangiabadi, Kouros Divsalar, Hossein Safizadeh, Zahra Esmaili, and Hossein Rafiei, "Effect of Prayer on Intensity of Migraine Headache: A Randomized Clinical Trial," *Journal of Evidence-Based Complementary and Alternative Medicine*, Feb. 2016, Vol. 22. No. 1.

37. Katja Wiech, Miguel Farias, Guy Kahane, Nicholas Shackel, Wiebke Tiede, and Irene Tracey, "An fMRI Study Measuring Analgesia Enhanced by Religion as a Belief System," *Pain*, Oct. 15, 2008, Vol. 139, Issue 2, pp. 467-476.

38. Interview of John Riccardo, "Unite Your Suffering to the Cross," YouTube, March 26, 2018, https://www.youtube.com/watch?v=Oi9-Q22o_es&t=606s.

39. "Most Americans Practice Charitable Giving, Volunteerism," Gallup, Dec. 13, 2013.

40. Robert D. Putnam and David E. Campbell, *American Grace: How Religion Divides and Unites Us*, Simon & Schuster, 2012, pp. 445-446.

41. Brett Pelham and Steve Crabtree, "Worldwide, Highly Religious More Likely to Help Others," Gallup, Oct. 8, 2008.

42. Eric S. Kim and Sara H. Konrath, "Volunteering is Prospectively Associated with Health Care Use Among Older Adults," *Social Science & Medicine*, Jan. 2016, Vol. 149, pp. 122-129.

43. Robert Grimm, Kimberly Spring, and Nathan Dietz, "The Health Benefits of Volunteering: A Review of Recent Research," April 2007, Corporation for National and Community Service.

44. Ibid.

45. Phyllis Moen, Donna Dempster-McClain, and Robin M. Williams, Jr., "Successful Aging: A Life-Course Perspective on Women's Multiple Roles and Health," *American Journal of Sociology*, May 1992, Vol. 97, No. 6, pp. 1612-1638.

46. Frank J. Infurna, Morris A. Okun, and Kevin J. Grimm, "Volunteering Is Associated with Lower Risk of Cognitive Impairment," *Journal of the American Geriatrics Society*, Oct. 2016, Vol. 64, No. 11.

47. Ellen J. Langer and Judith Rodin, "The Effects of Choice and Enhanced Personal Responsibility for the Aged: A Field Experiment in an Institutional Setting," *Journal of Personality and Social Psychology*, Sept. 1976, Vol. 34, Issue 2, pp. 191-198.

48. Phyllis Moen, Donna Dempster-McClain, and Robin M. Williams, Jr., "Successful Aging: A Life-Course Perspective on Women's Multiple Roles and Health," *American Journal of Sociology*, May 1992, Vol. 97, No. 6, pp. 1612-1638.

49. Robert Grimm, Kimberly Spring, and Nathan Dietz, "The Health Benefits of Volunteering: A Review of Recent Research," April 2007, Corporation for National and Community Service.

50. Lynda H. Powell, Leila Shahabi, and Carl E. Thoresen, "Religion and Spirituality: Linkages to Physical Health," *American Psychologist*, Jan. 2003, Vol. 58, No 1.

51. Marc A. Musick and John Wilson, "Volunteering and Depression: The Role of Psychological and Social Resources in Different Age Groups," *Social Science & Medicine*, Jan. 2003, Vol. 56, Issue 2, pp. 259-269.

52. Christopher G. Ellison and Linda K. George, "Religious Involvement, Social Ties, and Social Support in a Southeastern Community," *Journal for the Scientific Study of Religion*, 1994, Vol. 33, No. 1, pp. 46-61.

53. Neal Krause, "Church-Based Volunteering, Providing Informal Support at Church, and Self-Rated Health in Late Life," *Journal of Aging and Health*, March 2009, Vol. 21, No. 1, pp. 63-84.

Chapter 3: Belief Breeds Happiness

1. John Moran's answer to, "What is your worldview?," Quora.com, Jan. 23, 2019 and, "How did God change your life?," Quora.com, June 27, 2018, https://www. quora.com/What-is-your-worldview/answer/John-Moran-129; https://www.quora. com/How-did-God-change-your-life.

2. Steven Pirutinsky, Aaron D. Cherniak, and David H. Rosmarin, "COVID-19, Mental Health, and Religious Coping Among American Orthodox Jews," *Journal of Religion and Health*, July 2020, Vol. 59, pp. 2288-2301.

3. Ed Diener and Robert Biswas-Diener, *Happiness: Unlocking the Mysteries of Psychological Wealth*, Blackwell Publishing, 2008, p. 114.

4. Chaeyoon Lim and Robert D. Putnam, "Religion, Social Networks, and Life Satisfaction," *American Sociological Review*, Dec. 2010, Vol. 75, No. 6, pp. 914-933.

5. Cited in Jonathan Gruber, "Religious Market Structure, Religious Participation, and Outcomes: Is Religion Good for You?," National Bureau of Economic Research working paper 11377, May 2005.

6. "COVID 19, Religion and Health," YouTube, Sept. 29, 2020, https://www.youtube.com/watch?v=ZhJoWw1PMsc.

7. Harold Koenig, "Religion/Spirituality and Recovery from Mental Illness, Moral Injury and PTSD," YouTube, Sept. 26, 2020, www.youtube.com/watch?v=iejSPK-FNyc.

8. Ying Chen and Tyler J. VanderWeele, "Associations of Religious Upbringing With Subsequent Health and Well-Being From Adolescence to Young Adulthood: An Outcome-Wide Analysis," *American Journal of Epidemiology*, Sept. 2018, Vol. 187, No. 11.

9. Cited in Patrick F. Fagan, "Why Religion Matters Even More: The Impact of Religious Practice on Social Stability," Backgrounder, The Heritage Foundation, Dec. 18, 2006.

10. Ying Chen and Tyler J. VanderWeele, "Associations of Religious Upbringing With Subsequent Health and Well-Being From Adolescence to Young Adulthood: An Outcome-Wide Analysis," *American Journal of Epidemiology*, Sept. 2018, Vol. 187, No. 11.

11. Ed Diener and Robert Biswas-Diener, *Happiness: Unlocking the Mysteries of Psychological Wealth*, Blackwell Publishing, 2008, p. 114.

12. John F. Helliwell, Richard Layard, Jeffrey Sachs, Jan-Emmanuel De Neve, Lara B. Aknin, and Shun Wang, eds., *World Happiness Report 2021*, New York: Sustainable Development Solutions Network.

13. David Borovsky, "Are Scandinavians Really That Happy?", Foundation for Economic Education, FEE.org, Feb. 9, 2018, https://fee.org/articles/are-scandinavians-really-that-happy/.

14. Joey Marshall, "Are Religious People Happier, Healthier? Our New Global Study Explores This Question," FactTank, Pew Research Center, Jan. 31, 2019, https://pewrsr.ch/2MEWOYx.

15. "Religiosity, Income, Health and Life Satisfaction," *Crossroads*, newsletter of the Center for Spirituality, Theology, and Health, Duke University, Vol. 9, Issue 9, March 2020.

16. Paul Joydhar, "Testimony: My Life Since I Became A Christian," King James Bible Online, July 25, 2017, https://www.kingjamesbibleonline.org/testimony_my-life-since-i-became-a-christian/.

17. Robert Spitzer, "The Four Levels of Happiness," Spitzer Center for Visionary

Leadership, https://spitzercenter.org/what-we-do/educate/four-levels-of-happiness/.

18. Ibid.

19. C.S. Lewis, *Mere Christianity*, HarperCollins, 1952, p. 50.

20. Kath Koch, *Finding Authentic Hope and Wholeness: 5 Questions That Will Change Your Life*, Moody Publishers, 2005, p. 122. Also Arden Compton, "Antidote to the 7 P's of Pride," lessonsfromtheloaves.com, July 15, 2015, https://lessonsfromtheloaves. wordpress.com/2015/07/15/antidote-to-the-7-ps-of-pride-praise-power-profits-position-prestige-possessions-and-pleasure/.

21. Bob Unruh, "Dad Links Son's Suicide to 'The God Delusion', *World Net Daily*, Nov. 20, 2008.

22. Harold Koenig, "Religion, Spirituality, and Health: The Research and Clinical Implications," *ISRN Psychiatry*, Dec. 2012, Article ID 278730.

23. Colleen McClain-Jacobson, Barry Rosenfeld, Anne Kosinski, Hayley Pessin, James E. Cimino, and William Breitbart, "Belief in an Afterlife, Spiritual Well-Being and End-of-Life Despair in Patients with Advanced Cancer," *General Hospital Psychiatry*, 2004, Vol. 26, pp. 484-486.

24. Jeffrey Long, *Evidence of the Afterlife: The Science of Near-Death Experiences*, HarperOne, 2011.

25. "Dr. Harold Koenig Faith and Health," YouTube, Healthy Human Revolution channel, Jan. 28, 2019, https://www.youtube.com/watch?v=asS4gnu-aII.

26. "Looking for Satisfaction and Happiness in a Career? Start by Choosing a Job That Helps Others," National Opinion Research Center at the University of Chicago, *Science Daily*, April 19 2007, https://www.sciencedaily.com/releases/2007/04/070419092028.htm.

27. Genevieve Pollock, "Study Finds Most Catholic Priests are Happy, Appreciate Celibacy," Zenit News Agency, Oct. 9, 2011.

28. Jeff Levin, *God, Faith, and Health: Exploring the Spirituality-Healing Connection*, John Wiley & Sons, 2001, p. 26.

29. Mary Fairchild, "Read Short 'Popcorn' Testimonies of Transformed Lives," Learnreligions.com, March 19, 2018.

30. Rick Nauert, "Thinking of God Calms Believers, Stresses Atheists," *LiveScience*, August 5, 2010, https://www.livescience.com/8434-thinking-god-calms-believers-stresses-atheists.html.

31. Michael Inzlicht and Alexa M. Tullett, "Reflecting on God: Religious Primes Can Reduce Neurophysiological Response to Errors," *Psychological Science*, Aug. 2010, Vol. 21, No. 8., pp. 1184-1190.

32. Zeev Kaplan, Michael A. Matar, Ram Kamin, Tamar Sadan, and Hagit Cohen, "Stress-Related Responses After 3 Years of Exposure to Terror in Israel: Are Ideological-Religious Factors Associated With Resilience?," *The Journal of Clinical Psychiatry*, Oct. 2005, Vol. 66, Issue 9, pp. 1146-54.

33. "Effects of Religious Practice on Health," Marriage & Religion Research Institute, http://marripedia.org/effects_of_religious_practice_on_health.

34. Byron R. Johnson, Ralph Brett, and Derek Webb, *Objective Hope: Assessing the Effectiveness of Faith-Based Organizations*, Center for Research on Religion and Urban Civil Society, University of Pennsylvania, 2002.

35. Harold Koenig, "Religion, Spirituality, and Health: The Research and Clinical Implications," *ISRN Psychiatry*, Dec. 2012, Article ID 278730.

36. Howard M. Bahr and Bruce A. Chadwick, "Religion and Family in Middletown,

USA," *Journal of Marriage and Family*, May 1985, Vol. 47, No. 2, pp. 407-414.
37. Nathaniel M. Lambert, Frank D. Fincham, Scott R. Braithwaite, Steven M. Graham, and Steven R.H. Beach, "Can Prayer Increase Gratitude?," *Psychology of Religion and Spirituality*, 2009, Vol. 1, No. 3, pp. 139-149.
38. "Prayer, Gratitude, and Forgiveness," YouTube video, Feb. 9, 2021, https://www.youtube.com/watch?v=HmwOAl0PpbM.
39. Ed Diener and Robert Biswas-Diener, *Happiness: Unlocking the Mysteries of Psychological Wealth*, Blackwell Publishing, 2008, p. 115.
40. Ibid, p. 117.
41. Harold G. Koenig, *Is Religion Good for Your Health? The Effects of Religion on Physical and Mental Health*, The Haworth Pastoral Press, 1997, p. 67.
42. "Understanding the Instinctive Drive for Social Interactions," NOMIS Research Project, Harvard University (undated), https://nomisfoundation.ch/research-projects/understanding-the-instinctive-drive-for-social-interactions/.
43. Jeff Levin, *Religion and Medicine: A History of the Encounter Between Humanity's Two Greatest Institutions*, Oxford University Press, 2020, p. 89. Also: Jessica Morales, "The Heart's Electromagnetic Field Is Your Superpower," *Psychology Today*, Nov. 29, 2020.
44. Harold Koenig, "Religion/Spirituality and Recovery from Mental Illness, Moral Injury and PTSD," YouTube, Sept. 26, 2020, https://www.youtube.com/watch?v=ie-jSPK-FNyc.

Chapter 4: Defeating Depression, Drugs, and Drink

1. Cited in Harold G. Koenig, Michael E. McCullough, and David B. Larson, *Handbook of Religion and Health*, Oxford University Press, 2001, p. 58.
2. "Mental Health By the Numbers," National Alliance on Mental Illness, https://nami.org/mhstats; "Mental Health Disorder Statistics," Johns Hopkins Medicine, https://www.hopkinsmedicine.org/health/wellness-and-prevention/mental-health-disorder-statistics.
3. "Key Substance Use and Mental Health Indicators in the United States: Results from the 2019 National Survey on Drug Use and Health," Substance Abuse and Mental Health Services Administration (SAMHSA), U.S. Department of Health and Human Services, Sept. 2020, pp. 42-44.
4. "The Impact of COVID-19 on Pediatric Mental Health: A Study of Private Healthcare Claims," FAIR Health white paper, March 2, 2021.
5. Jean M. Twenge, A. Bell Cooper, Thomas E. Joiner, Mary E. Duffy, and Sarah G. Binau, "Age, Period, and Cohort Trends in Mood Disorder Indicators and Suicide-Related Outcomes in a Nationally Representative Dataset, 2005-2017," *Journal of Abnormal Psychology*, 2019, Vol. 128, No. 3, 185-199.
6. Jeffrey M. Jones, "U.S. Church Membership Falls Below Majority for First Time," Gallup, March 29, 2021, https://news.gallup.com/poll/341963/church-membership-falls-below-majority-first-time.aspx.
7. Pew Research, "Trends in Religious Composition of U.S. Adults" detailed tables, https://www.pewforum.org/2019/10/17/in-u-s-decline-of-christianity-continues-at-rapid-pace/; https://www.pewforum.org/wp-content/uploads/sites/7/2019/10/Detailed-Tables-v1-FOR-WEB.pdf.
8. Aleaya Bella, "My Testimony. How Jesus Saved Me from Depression and Anxiety," YouTube, Feb. 8, 2021, https://youtu.be/9IiwnAW3YXE.
9. Shane Sharp, "How Does Prayer Help Manage Emotions?," *Social Psychology*

Quarterly, Dec. 2010, Vol. 73, No. 4, pp. 417-437.

10. Andrew Stern, "Study Links Religious Services to Optimism," Reuters, Nov. 10, 2011.

11. Frank Newport, Sangeeta Agrawal, and Dan Witters, "Very Religious Americans Report Less Depression, Worry," Gallup, Dec. 1, 2010.

12. Tyler J. VanderWeele, "Religion and Health: A Synthesis," In: Peteet, J.R. and Balboni, M.J. (Eds.), *Spirituality and Religion within the Culture of Medicine: From Evidence to Practice*. New York, NY: Oxford University Press, 2017.

13. Byron R. Johnson, Ralph Brett, and Derek Webb, *Objective Hope: Assessing the Effectiveness of Faith-Based Organizations*, Center for Research on Religion and Urban Civil Society, University of Pennsylvania, 2002.

14. Harold Koenig, "Religion, Spirituality, and Health: The Research and Clinical Implications," *ISRN Psychiatry*, Dec. 2012, Article ID 278730.

15. Fatemeh Marashian and Elahe Esmaili, "Relationship Between Religious Beliefs of Students with Mental Health Disorders Among the Students of Islamic Azad University of Ahvaz," *Procedia—Social and Behavioral Sciences*, 2012, Vol. 46, pp. 1831-1833.

16. Harold G. Koenig and Saad Saleh Al Shohaib, "Religiosity and Mental Health in Islam," in H.S. Moffic, J.R. Peteet, A. Hankir, and R Awaad, Eds., *Islamophobia and Psychiatry: Recognition, Prevention, and Treatment*, 2018, pp. 55-65.

17. Brian Walsh, "Does Spirituality Make You Happy?," *Time*, Aug. 7, 2017.

18. Harold G. Koenig, Linda K. George, and Bercedis L. Peterson, "Religiosity and Remission of Depression in Medically Ill Older Patients," *American Journal of Psychiatry*, April 1998, Vol. 155, Issue 4, pp. 536-542.

19. "Having Religious Faith Can Speed Recovery From Depression In Older Patients, *Science Daily*, May 4, 1998.

20. Claire Gecewicz, "Few Americans Say Their House of Worship is Open, but a Quarter Say Their Faith Has Grown Amid Pandemic," April 30, 2020, Pew Research Center, https://www.pewresearch.org/fact-tank/2020/04/30/few-americans-say-their-house-of-worship-is-open-but-a-quarter-say-their-religious-faith-has-grown-amid-pandemic/.

21. G. Lucchetti, L.G. Góes, S.G. Amaral, G. Ganadjian, I. Andrade, P.O. de Araújo Almeida, and M.E.G. Manso, "Spirituality, Religiosity and the Mental Health Consequences of Social Isolation During Covid-19 Pandemic," *International Journal of Social Psychiatry*, Nov. 2020.

22. "Mental Health in Congregations Study," Department of Sociology, The Catholic University of America, https://sociology.catholic.edu/mental-health-congregations/index.html.

23. Ellen L. Idler and Stanislav V. Kasl, "Religion Among Disabled and Nondisabled Persons II: Attendance at Religious Services as a Predictor of the Course of Disability," *Journal of Gerontology Series B*, Dec. 1997, Vol. 52B, No. 6, pp. S306-S316.

24. Kenneth I. Pargament, Bruce W. Smith, Harold G. Koenig, and Lisa Perez, "Patterns of Positive and Negative Religious Coping with Major Life Stressors," *Journal for the Scientific Study of Religion*, Dec., 1998, Vol. 37, No. 4, pp. 710-724.

25. Harold Koenig, Kenneth I. Pargament, and Julie Nielsen, "Religious Coping and Health Status in Medically Ill Hospitalized Older Adults," *Journal of Nervous and Mental Disease*, Sept. 1998, Vol. 186, Issue 9, pp. 513-521.

26. David H. Rosmarin and Bethany Leidl, "Spirituality, Religion, and Anxiety

Disorders," in *Handbook of Spirituality, Religion, and Mental Health,* second edition, David H. Rosmarin and Harold G. Koenig (Eds.), Academic Press, an imprint of Elsevier, 2020, p. 46.

27. Andrew Newberg, "How God Changes Your Brain: An Introduction to Jewish Neurotheology," *CCAR Journal: The Reform Jewish Quarterly,* Winter 2016.

28. National Public Radio interview of Dr. Andrew Newberg, "Neuro-theology: This Is Your Brain On Religion," Dec. 15, 2010. https://www.npr.org/2010/12/15/132078267/neurotheology-where-religion-and-science-collide.

29. Lisa Miller, Ravi Bansal, Priya Wickramaratne, Xuejun Hao, Craig E. Tenke, Myrna M. Weissman, and Bradley S. Peterson, "Neuroanatomical Correlates of Religiosity and Spirituality: A Study in Adults at High and Low Familial Risk for Depression," *JAMA Psychiatry,* 2014, Vol. 71, No. 2, pp. 128-135.

30. Loyd S. Wright, Christopher J. Frost, and Stephen J. Wisecarver, "Church Attendance, Meaningfulness of Religion, and Depressive Symptomatology Among Adolescents," *Journal of Youth and Adolescence,* 1993, Vol. 22, No. 5.

31. Patrick F. Fagan, "Why Religion Matters: The Impact of Religious Practice on Social Stability," Backgrounder, The Heritage Foundation, Jan. 25, 1996.

32. Frank Newport, Sangeeta Agrawal, and Dan Witters, "Very Religious Americans Report Less Depression, Worry," Gallup, Dec. 1, 2010.

33. Tyler J. VanderWeele, "Religion and Health: A Synthesis," In: Peteet, J.R. and Balboni, M.J. (Eds.), *Spirituality and Religion within the Culture of Medicine: From Evidence to Practice,* Oxford University Press, 2017.

34. Ann Marie Sorenson, Carl F. Grindstaff, and R. Jay Turner, "Religious Involvement Among Unmarried Adolescent Mothers: A Source of Emotional Support?," *Sociology of Religion,* Spring 1995, Vol. 56, No. 1, pp. 71-81.

35. Mary Cuadrado and Louis Lieberman, "The Virgin of Guadalupe as an Ancillary Modality for Treating Hispanic Substance Abusers: Juramentos in the United States," *Journal of Religion and Health,* Nov. 2009, Vol. 50, Issue 4, pp. 922-30.

36. Samuel G. Freedman, "Alcoholics Anonymous, Without the Religion," *New York Times,* Feb. 21, 2014.

37. Sources: National Institute on Alcohol Abuse and Alcoholism, National Center for Health Statistics, Centers for Disease Control, https://wonder.cdc.gov/.

38. Mary Fairchild, "Read Short 'Popcorn' Testimonies of Transformed Lives," Learnreligions.com, March 19, 2018.

39. Patrick F. Fagan, "Why Religion Matters Even More: The Impact of Religious Practice on Social Stability," Backgrounder, The Heritage Foundation, Dec. 18, 2006.

40. Harold Koenig, "Religion, Spirituality, and Health: The Research and Clinical Implications," *ISRN Psychiatry,* Dec. 2012, Article ID 278730.

41. Patrick F. Fagan, "Why Religion Matters: The Impact of Religious Practice on Social Stability," Backgrounder, The Heritage Foundation, Jan. 25, 1996.

42. Michael N. Dohn, Santa Altagracia Jiménez Méndez, Maximinia Nolasco Pozo, Elizabet Altagracia Cabrera, and Anita L. Dohn, "Alcohol Use and Church Attendance Among Seventh Through Twelfth Grade Students, Dominican Republic," *Journal of Religion and Health,* Nov. 2012, Vol. 53, Issue 3, pp. 675-689.

43. Patrick F. Fagan, "Why Religion Matters Even More: The Impact of Religious Practice on Social Stability," Backgrounder, The Heritage Foundation, Dec. 18, 2006.

44. Ibid.

45. Ying Chen, Howard K. Koh, Ichiro Kawachi, Michael Botticelli, and Tyler

VanderWeele, "Religious Service Attendance and Deaths Related to Drugs, Alcohol, and Suicide Among US Health Care Professionals," *JAMA Psychiatry*, July 1, 2020, Vol. 77, No. 1, pp. 737-744.

Chapter 5: Church Cultivates Integrity and Self-Discipline

1. Jonah Goldberg, *The Suicide of the West*, Crown Forum, 2018, p. 333.
2. John Bingham, "Richard Dawkins: I Can't Be Sure God Does Not Exist," *The Telegraph*, Feb. 24, 2012.
3. Jonathon Van Maren, "Atheists Sound the Alarm: Decline of Christianity is Seriously Hurting Society," *LifeSiteNews*, Nov. 4, 2019.
4. Jesse M. Bering, Katrina McLeod, and Todd K. Shackelford, "Reasoning About Dead Agents Reveals Possible Adaptive Trends," *Human Nature*, Winter 2005, Vol. 16, No. 4, pp. 360-381.
5. Jared Piazza, Jesse M. Bering, and Gordon Ingram, "'Princess Alice is Watching You': Children's Belief in an Invisible Person Inhibits Cheating," *Journal of Experimental Child Psychology*, Vol. 109, Issue 3, July 2011, pp. 311-320.
6. Alex Spiegel, "Is Believing In God Evolutionarily Advantageous?," National Public Radio, Aug. 30, 2010.
7. Azim F. Shariff and Ara Norenzayan, "Mean Gods Make Good People: Different Views of God Predict Cheating Behavior," *International Journal for the Psychology of Religion*, 2011, Vol. 21, Issue 2.
8. Audio remarks by Azam Shariff, "Different Views of God May Influence Academic Cheating," University of Oregon press release and audio clips, April 20, 2011, https://uonews.uoregon.edu/archive/news-release/2011/4/different-views-god-may-influence-academic-cheating
9. "The Eleven Voluntary Initiatives of Ted Turner," Jotman.com, Nov. 1, 2008, https://jotman.blogspot.com/2008/11/eleven-voluntary-initiatives-of-ted.html.
10. Michael E. McCullough and Brian L.B. Willoughby, "Religion, Self-Regulation, and Self-Control: Associations, Explanations, and Implications," *Psychological Bulletin*, 2009, Vol. 135, No. 1, pp. 69-93.
11. Kristin Laurin, Aaron C. Kay, and Gráinne M. Fitzsimons, "Divergent Effects of Activating Thoughts of God on Self-Regulation," *Journal of Personality and Social Psychology*, 2012, Vol. 102, No. 1, pp. 4-21.
12. June P. Tangney, Roy F. Baumeister, and Angie Luzio Boone, "High Self-Control Predicts Good Adjustment, Less Pathology, Better Grades, and Interpersonal Success," *Journal of Personality*, April 2004, Vol. 72, No. 2, 271-322.
13. Angela L. Duckworth and Martin E.P. Seligman, "Self-Discipline Outdoes IQ in Predicting Academic Performance of Adolescents," *Psychological Science*, Dec. 2005, Vol. 16, No. 12, pp. 939-944.
14. Michael E. McCullough and Brian L.B. Willoughby, "Religion, Self-Regulation, and Self-Control: Associations, Explanations, and Implications," *Psychological Bulletin*, 2009, Vol. 135, No. 1, pp. 69-93.
15. "Self-Control," *Psychology Today*, https://www.psychologytoday.com/us/basics/self-control.
16. Patrick McNamara, "The Motivational Origins of Religious Practices," *Zygon: Journal of Religion and Science*, Jan. 2004, Vol. 37, No. 1, pp. 143-160.
17. Michael E. McCullough and Brian L.B. Willoughby, "Religion, Self-Regulation, and Self-Control: Associations, Explanations, and Implications," *Psychological Bulle-*

tin, 2009, Vol. 135, No. 1, 69-93.

18. Kristin Laurin, Aaron C. Kay, and Gráinne M. Fitzsimons. "Divergent Effects of Activating Thoughts of God on Self-Regulation," *Journal of Personality and Social Psychology*, Oct. 2011, Vol. 102, No. 1, 4-21.

19. Ibid.

20. Bengi Öner-Özkan, "Future Time Orientation and Religion," *Social Behavior and Personality: An International Journal*, Jan. 2007, Vol. 35, No. 1, pp. 51-62.

21. Doran C. French, Nancy Eisenberg, Julie Vaughan, Urip Purwono, and Telie A. Suryanti, "Religious Involvement and the Social Competence and Adjustment of Indonesian Muslim Adolescents," *Developmental Psychology*, March 2008, Vol. 44, No. 2, 597-611.

22. Shagufta Aziz and Ghazala Rehman, "Self-Control and Tolerance Among Low and High Religious Groups," *Journal of Personality and Clinical Studies*, 1996, Vol. 12, No. 1-2, pp. 83-85.

23. Kevin Rounding, Albert Lee, Jill A. Jacobson, and Li-Jun Ji, "Religion Replenishes Self-Control," *Psychological Science*, May 2012, Vol. 23, No. 6, 635-642.

24. Justin Marc David Harrison and Ryan Thomas McKay, "Do Religious and Moral Concepts Influence the Ability to Delay Gratification? A Priming Study," *Journal of Articles in Support of the Null Hypothesis*, 2013, Vol. 10, No. 1.

25. Michael E. McCullough and Brian L.B. Willoughby, "Religion, Self-Regulation, and Self-Control: Associations, Explanations, and Implications," *Psychological Bulletin*, 2009, Vol. 135, No. 1, pp. 69-93.

26. Scott A. Desmond, "Secrets and Lies: Adolescent Religiosity and Concealing Information from Parents," *Religions*, Feb. 2019, Vol. 10, No. 2, 132.

27. Michael E. McCullough and Brian L.B. Willoughby, "Religion, Self-Regulation, and Self-Control: Associations, Explanations, and Implications," *Psychological Bulletin*, 2009, Vol. 135, No. 1, pp. 69-93.

28. Kristin Laurin, Aaron C. Kay, and Gráinne M. Fitzsimons. "Divergent Effects of Activating Thoughts of God on Self-Regulation," *Journal of Personality and Social Psychology*, Oct. 2011, Vol. 102, No. 1, 4-21.

29. Edward Alsworth Ross, *Sin and Society: An Analysis of Latter-Day Iniquity*, Houghton, Mifflin, Boston and New York, 1907. (Kindle edition)

30. Denali Tietjen, "Men Who Watch Pornography Have Small Brains," Boston. com, May 30, 2014, https://www.boston.com/culture/health/2014/05/30/men-who-watch-pornography-have-small-brains.

31. Everett L. Worthington Jr., Kevin Bursley, James T. Berry, Michael McCullough, Sasha N. Baier, Jack W. Berry, Nathaniel G. Wade, and David E. Canter, "Religious Commitment, Religious Experiences, and Ways of Coping With Sexual Attraction," *Marriage & Family: A Christian Journal*, Jan. 2001, Vol. 4, No. 4, pp. 411-423.

32. Mary B. Short, Thomas E. Kasper, and Chad T. Wetterneck, "The Relationship Between Religiosity and Internet Pornography Use," *Journal of Religion and Health*, April 2015, Vol. 54, No. 2, pp. 571-583.

33. Joseph Tkach, "Christian Living: How to Resist Temptation," Grace Communion International, gci.org, https://www.gci.org/articles/how-to-resist-temptation/

Chapter 6: Couples Who Pray Together Stay Together

1. David Housholder, "7 Secrets to a Long and Strong Marriage. Our 39th anniversary today.", YouTube, Jan. 9, 2021, https://youtu.be/__Nm4u8GByU.

2. Brian Hollar, "Regular Church Attenders Marry More and Divorce Less Than Their Less Devout Peers," Institute for Family Studies blog, March 4, 2020.

3. Chris M. Wilson and Andrew J. Oswald, How Does Marriage Affect Physical and Psychological Health? A Survey of the Longitudinal Evidence, June 2005, IZA Bonn Discussion Paper No. 1619, The Institute for the Study of Labor.

4. Howard S. Friedman and Leslie R. Martin, *The Longevity Project*, Penguin Group, 2012, p. 117.

5. Tyler VanderWeele, "What the New York Times Gets Wrong About Marriage, Health, and Well-Being," Institute for Family Studies blog, May 13, 2017, https://ifstudies.org/blog/what-the-new-york-times-gets-wrong-about-marriage-health-and-well-being.

6. Shawn Grover and John F. Helliwell, "How's Life at Home? New Evidence on Marriage and the Set Point for Happiness," *Journal of Happiness Studies*, Feb. 2019, Vol. 20, Issue 2.

7. Robert G. Wood, Brian Goesling, and Sarah Avellar, "The Effects of Marriage on Health: A Synthesis of Recent Research Evidence," Mathematica Policy Research Inc., June 19, 2007.

8. Alice G. Walton, "The Marriage Problem: Why Many Are Choosing Cohabitation Instead," *The Atlantic*, Feb. 7, 2012.

9. W. Bradford Wilcox and Nicholas H. Wolfinger, "Then Comes Marriage? Religion, Race, and Marriage in Urban America," *Social Science Research*, June 2007, Vol. 36, Issue 2.

10. "Ephraim + Sussie | 25 Years of Marriage," YouTube, July 7, 2017, https://youtu.be/YHePURRciAY.

11. Frank D. Fincham and Steven R.H. Beach, "I Say a Little Prayer for You: Praying for Partner Increases Commitment in Romantic Relationships, *Journal of Family Psychology*, 2014, Vol. 28, No. 5.

12. Brandon Showalter, "Married Couples Who Attend Church Services Together Are Less Likely to Divorce: Study," *Christian Post*, Dec. 2, 2016, https://www.christianpost.com/news/married-couples-who-attend-church-services-together-are-less-likely-to-divorce-study.html.

13. Ibid.

14. Cited in Patrick F. Fagan, "Why Religion Matters Even More: The Impact of Religious Practice on Social Stability," Backgrounder, The Heritage Foundation, Dec. 18, 2006.

15. "Effects of Religious Practice on Marriage," Marripedia, Marriage and Religion Research Institute, http://marripedia.org/effects_of_religious_practice_on_marriage.

16. Jason S. Carroll, Laurie DeRose, David C. Dollahite, Spencer L. James, Byron R. Johnson, Loren Marks, Richard Reeves, Wendy Wang, and W. Bradford Wilcox, "Faith, Feminism, and Marriage: Institutions, Norms, and Relationship Quality," *World Family Map 2019: Mapping Family Change and Child Well-Being Outcomes*, Institute for Family Studies, 2019, p. 22; "Effects of Religious Practice on Marriage," Marripedia, Marriage and Religion Research Institute, http://marripedia.org/effects_of_religious_practice_on_marriage.

17. Jason S. Carroll, Laurie DeRose, David C. Dollahite, Spencer L. James, Byron R. Johnson, Loren Marks, Richard Reeves, Wendy Wang, and W. Bradford Wilcox, "Faith, Feminism, and Marriage: Institutions, Norms, and Relationship Quality," *World Family Map 2019: Mapping Family Change and Child Well-Being Outcomes*, Institute for Family Studies, 2019, pp. 22-24.

18. Howard M. Bahr and Bruce A. Chadwick, "Religion and Family in Middletown, USA," *Journal of Marriage and Family*, May 1985, Vol. 47, No. 2.

19. Vaughn R. A. Call and Tim B. Heaton, "Religious Influence on Marital Stability," *Journal for the Scientific Study of Religion*, Sept. 1997, Vol. 36, No. 3, pp. 382-392.

20. W. Bradford Wilcox and Nicholas H. Wolfinger, "Better Together: Religious Attendance, Gender, and Relationship Quality," Institute for Family Studies, ifstudies.org, Feb. 11, 2016, https://ifstudies.org/blog/better-together-religious-attendance-gender-and-relationship-quality.

21. W. Bradford Wilcox, *Soft Patriarchs, New Men: How Christianity Shapes Fathers and Husbands*, University of Chicago Press, 2004, p. 186. Cited in https://www.nationalreview.com/2016/02/religious-attendance-improves-relationships/.

22. Cited in Patrick F. Fagan, "Why Religion Matters Even More: The Impact of Religious Practice on Social Stability," Backgrounder, The Heritage Foundation, Dec. 18, 2006.

23. Adelle M. Banks, "Research Disputes 'Facts' on Christian Divorces," *The Christian Century*, March 14, 2011.

24. Quoted in Adelle M. Banks, Religion News Service, March 25, 2011.

25. "Divorce (Still) Less Likely Among Catholics," 1964, a research blog for the Center for Applied Research in the Apostolate, Sept. 26, 2013, http://nineteensixty-four.blogspot.com/2013/09/divorce-still-less-likely-among.html.

26. David C. Atkins and Deborah E. Kessel, "Religiousness and Infidelity: Attendance, but Not Faith and Prayer, Predict Marital Fidelity," *Journal of Marriage and Family*, May, 2008, Vol. 70, No. 2.

27. "American Catholics Clash With Church Over 'Sins,' Survey Finds," NBCnews.com, Sept. 2, 2015, https://www.nbcnews.com/news/us-news/american-catholics-clash-church-over-sins-survey-finds-n419406.

28. Richard J. Fehring and Michael D. Manhart, "Natural Family Planning and Marital Chastity: The Effects of Periodic Abstinence on Marital Relationships," *The Linacre Quarterly*, June 2020.

29. Mercedes Arzú Wilson, "The Practice of Natural Family Planning Versus the Use of Artificial Birth Control: Family, Sexual, and Moral Issues," *Catholic Social Science Review*, 2002, Vol. 7, pp. 185-211, http://lifeissues.net/writers/wils/wils_01naturalfamilyplanning2.html.

30. Annette Mahoney, Kenneth I. Pargament, Nichole Murray-Swank, and Aaron Murray-Swank, "Religion and the Sanctification of Family Relationships," *Review of Religious Research*, March 2003, Vol. 44, No. 3, p. 220.

31. W. Bradford Wilcox and Nicholas H. Wolfinger, "Then Comes Marriage? Religion, Race, and Marriage in Urban America," *Social Science Research*, June 2007, Vol. 36, No. 2.

32. Ed Stetzer, "One-on-One with Tony Merida on Christ-Centered Conflict Resolution," The Exchange with Ed Stetzer, *Christianity Today*, June 23, 2020, https://www.christianitytoday.com/edstetzer/2020/june/one-on-one-with-tony-merida-on-christ-centered-conflict-res.html.

33. Frank D. Fincham and Steven R.H. Beach, "I Say a Little Prayer for You: Praying for Partner Increases Commitment in Romantic Relationships, *Journal of Family Psychology*, 2014, Vol. 28, No. 5.

34. Ross W. May, Ashley N. Cooper, and Frank D. Fincham, "Prayer in Marriage to

Improve Wellness: Relationship Quality and Cardiovascular Functioning," *Journal of Religion and Health*, Dec. 2020, Vol. 59, No. 6, pp. 2990-3003.

35. Christopher G. Ellison, Andrea K. Henderson, Norval D. Glenn, and Kristine E. Harkrider, "Sanctification, Stress, and Marital Quality," *Family Relations*, Oct. 2011, Vol. 60, Issue 4.

36. Carle Zimmerman, "Family Influence Upon Religion," *Journal of Comparative Family Studies*, Autumn 1974, Vol. 5, No. 2.

37. Christopher G. Ellison, Andrea K. Henderson, Norval D. Glenn, and Kristine E. Harkrider, "Sanctification, Stress, and Marital Quality," *Family Relations*, Oct. 2011, Vol. 60, Issue 4.

38. Annette Mahoney, Kenneth I. Pargament, Nichole Murray-Swank, and Aaron Murray-Swank, "Religion and the Sanctification of Family Relationships," *Review of Religious Research*, March 2003, Vol. 44, No. 3, p. 220.

39. Frank D. Fincham and Steven R.H. Beach, "Marriage in the New Millennium: A Decade in Review," *Journal of Marriage and Family*, June 2010, Vol. 72, Issue 3, pp. 630-649.

40. Annette Mahoney, Kenneth I. Pargament, Tracey Jewell, and Aaron B. Swank, "Marriage and the Spiritual Realm: The Role of Proximal and Distal Religious Constructs in Marital Functioning," *Journal of Family Psychology*, Sept. 1999, Vol. 13, No. 3.

41. Christopher G. Ellison, Andrea K. Henderson, Norval D. Glenn, and Kristine E. Harkrider, "Sanctification, Stress, and Marital Quality," *Family Relations*, Oct. 2011, Vol. 60, Issue 4, pp. 404-420.

42. Ibid.

43. Patrick F. Fagan, "Why Religion Matters: The Impact of Religious Practice on Social Stability," Backgrounder, The Heritage Foundation, Jan. 25, 1996.

44. Jason S. Carroll, Laurie DeRose, David C. Dollahite, Spencer L. James, Byron R. Johnson, Loren Marks, Richard Reeves, Wendy Wang, and W. Bradford Wilcox, "Faith, Feminism, and Marriage: Institutions, Norms, and Relationship Quality," *World Family Map 2019: Mapping Family Change and Child Well-Being Outcomes*, Institute for Family Studies, 2019, p. 22.

45. Margot Cleveland, "Why Practicing Catholics Definitely Have the Best Sex," *The Federalist*, April 5, 2017.

46. Will Wright, "What Practicing NFP is Like: One Man Shares His Thoughts," CatholicLink, undated, https://catholic-link.org/what-nfp-is-like-male-perspective/.

47. "Humanae Vitae," encyclical of Pope Paul VI, July 25, 1968. The Vatican.

48. Cited in Patrick F. Fagan, "Why Religion Matters Even More: The Impact of Religious Practice on Social Stability," Backgrounder, The Heritage Foundation, Dec. 18, 2006.

49. Michael J. Rosenfeld and Katharina Roesler, "Cohabitation Experience and Cohabitation's Association With Marital Dissolution," *Journal of Marriage and Family*, Sept. 2018, Vol. 81, Issue 1.

50. Arland Thornton, William G. Axinn, and Daniel H. Hill, "Reciprocal Effects of Religiosity, Cohabitation, and Marriage," *American Journal of Sociology*, Nov., 1992, Vol. 98, No. 3.

51. Chris M. Wilson and Andrew J. Oswald, How Does Marriage Affect Physical and Psychological Health? A Survey of the Longitudinal Evidence, June 2005, IZA Bonn Discussion Paper No. 1619, The Institute for the Study of Labor.

52. "Why Marriage Matters, Third Edition: Thirty Conclusions from the Social Sciences," Institute for American Values, National Marriage Project, 2011, p. 6, 8.

Chapter 7: Faith Fosters Strong Families

1. "Six Secrets of Strong Families," condensed from Secrets of Strong Families by Nick Stinnett and John DeFrain, Everyday Enlightenment blog, http://willyac.word-press.com/everyday-articles/six-secrets-of-strong-families/.
2. Martin A. Johnson, "Family Life and Religious Commitment," *Review of Religious Research*, Spring 1973, Vol. 14, No. 3.
3. Sabrina McLuhan, "Traits of a Healthy Family," *The Interim*, April 25, 1984, http://www.theinterim.com/issues/marriage-family/traits-of-a-healthy-family-2/.
4. Lisa D. Pearce and William G. Axinn, "The Impact of Family Religious Life on the Quality of Mother-Child Relations," *American Sociological Review*, Dec. 1998, Vol. 63, No. 6.
5. Ibid.
6. Ibid.
7. W. Bradford Wilcox, *Soft Patriarchs, New Men: How Christianity Shapes Fathers and Husbands*, University of Chicago Press, 2004.
8. W. Bradford Wilcox, "Is Religion an Answer? Marriage, Fatherhood, and the Male Problematic," Research Brief No. 11, June 2008, Center for Marriage and Families, Institute for American Values.
9. Valarie King, "The Influence of Religion on Fathers' Relationships with Their Children," *Journal of Marriage and Family*, May 2003, Vol. 65, No. 2.
10. "The Value of Sit Down Family Meals for Emotional Health," eatingdisorder-hope.com, and Erica Jackson Curran, "7 Unexpected Benefits of Eating Together as a Family, According to Science," *Parents*, March 15, 2019, https://www.eatingdis-orderhope.com/blog/value-sit-down-family-meals-emotional-health, https://www.parents.com/recipes/tips/unexpected-benefits-of-eating-together-as-a-family-according-to-science/.
11. V. A. Krokonko, "The Spiritual Journey of a Single Parent," *Studies in Formative Spirituality*, 1986, Vol. 7, pp. 45-62, cited in Annette Mahoney, Kenneth I. Pargament, Nichole Murray-Swank, and Aaron Murray-Swank, "Religion and the Sanctification of Family Relationships," *Review of Religious Research*, March 2003, Vol. 44, No. 3, pp. 220-236.
12. Annette Mahoney, Kenneth I. Pargament, Nichole Murray-Swank, and Aaron Murray-Swank, "Religion and the Sanctification of Family Relationships," *Review of Religious Research*, March 2003, Vol. 44, No. 3, pp. 220-236.
13. Ibid.
14. S. Michael Craven, "Fathers: Key to Their Children's Faith," *The Christian Post*, June 19, 2011, https://www.christianpost.com/news/fathers-key-to-their-childrens-faith-51331/.
15. Brian L. McPhail, "Religious Heterogamy and the Intergenerational Transmission of Religion: A Cross-National Analysis," *Religions*, Feb. 2019, Vol. 10, Issue 2, p. 109.

Chapter 8: Church is Good for Kids

1. Ilana M. Horwitz, "The Abider-Avoider Achievement Gap: The Association Between GPA and Religiosity in Public Schools," Working Paper, March 2018.

2. Cited in Jonathan Gruber, "Religious Market Structure, Religious Participation, and Outcomes: Is Religion Good for You?," National Bureau of Economic Research working paper 11377, May 2005.

3. H. Hartshorne, M.A. May, and J.B. Maller, Studies in the Nature of Character: Vol. 2. Studies in Service and Self-Control, New York: Macmillan, 1929, cited in Michael E. McCullough and Brian L.B. Willoughby, "Religion, Self-Regulation, and Self-Control: Associations, Explanations, and Implications," *Psychological Bulletin*, 2009, Vol. 135, No. 1, pp. 69-93.

4. June P. Tangney, Roy F. Baumeister, and Angie Luzio Boone, "High Self-Control Predicts Good Adjustment, Less Pathology, Better Grades, and Interpersonal Success," *Journal of Personality*, April 2004, Vol. 72, No. 2, pp. 271-322.

5. Scott A. Desmond, Jeffery T. Ulmer, and Christopher D. Bader, "Religion, Self Control, and Substance Use," *Deviant Behavior*, Jan. 2013, Vol. 34, No. 5, pp. 384-406.

6. John P. Bartkowski, Xiaohe Xu, and Martin L. Levin, "Religion and Child Development: Evidence from the Early Childhood Longitudinal Study," *Social Science Research*, March 2008, Vol. 36, No 1, pp. 18-36.

7. Harold Koenig, "Religion/Spirituality and Recovery from Mental Illness, Moral Injury and PTSD," YouTube, Sept. 26, 2020, https://www.youtube.com/watch?v=ie-jSPK-FNyc.

8. Yuichi Shoda, Walter Mischel, and Philip K. Peake, "Predicting Adolescent Cognitive and Self-Regulatory Competencies from Preschool Delay of Gratification: Identifying Diagnostic Conditions," *Developmental Psychology*, 1990, Vol. 26, No. 6, pp. 978-986.

9. Angela L. Duckworth and Martin E.P. Seligman, "Self-Discipline Outdoes IQ in Predicting Academic Performance of Adolescents," *Psychological Science*, Dec. 2005, Vol. 16, No. 12, pp. 939-944.

10. The five "A's" are from Lisa Pearce's and Melinda Lundquist Denton's *A Faith of Their Own: Stability and Change in the Religiosity of America's Adolescents*, Oxford University Press, 2011.

11. "Effects of Religious Practice on Education," Marripedia, Marriage and Religion Research Institute, http://marripedia.org/effects_of_religious_practice_on_education.

12. Mark D. Regnerus, "Shaping School Success: Religious Socialization and Educational Outcomes in Metropolitan Public Schools," *Journal for the Scientific Study of Religion*, Sept. 2000, Vol. 39, No. 3.

13. Chandra Muller and Christopher G. Ellison, "Religious Involvement, Social Capital, and Adolescents' Academic Progress: Evidence From the National Education Longitudinal Study of 1988," *Sociological Focus*, May 2001, Vol. 34, No. 2, pp. 155-183.

14. Sandra L. Hanson and Alan L. Ginsburg, "Gaining Ground: Values and High School Success," *American Educational Research Journal*, Autumn 1988, Vol. 25, No. 3.

15. Chandra Muller and Christopher G. Ellison, "Religious Involvement, Social Capital, and Adolescents' Academic Progress: Evidence from the National Education Longitudinal Study of 1988," *Sociological Focus*, May 2001, Vol. 34, No. 2, pp. 155-183.

16. Christian Smith, "Research Note: Religious Participation and Parental Moral Expectations and Supervision of American Youth," *Review of Religious Research*, June 2003, Vol. 44, No. 4.

Holy Health

17. "Effects of Religious Practice on Education," Marripedia, Marriage and Religion Research Institute (undated), http://marripedia.org/effects_of_religious_practice_on_education.

18. Elaine Howard Ecklund and Kristen Schultz Lee, "Atheists and Agnostics Negotiate Religion and Family," *Journal for the Scientific Study of Religion*, Dec. 2011, Vol. 50, No. 4, pp. 728-743.

19. Jennifer L. Glanville, David Sikkink, and Edwin I. Hernández, "Religious Involvement and Educational Outcomes: The Role of Social Capital and Extracurricular Participation," *The Sociological Quarterly*, Winter 2008, Vol. 49, No. 1.

20. Michael Gottfried and Jacob Kirksey, "Self-Discipline and Catholic Schools: Evidence from Two National Cohorts," May 2018, published by the Thomas B. Fordham Institute.

21. William H. Jeynes, "A Meta-Analysis on the Effects and Contributions of Public, Public Charter, and Religious Schools on Student Outcomes," *Peabody Journal of Education*, 2012, Vol. 87, No. 3, pp. 305-335.

22. Michael Gottfried and Jacob Kirksey, "Self-Discipline and Catholic Schools: Evidence from Two National Cohorts," May 2018, published by the Thomas B. Fordham Institute.

23. William H. Jeynes, "A Meta-Analysis on the Effects and Contributions of Public, Public Charter, and Religious Schools on Student Outcomes," *Peabody Journal of Education*, 2012, Vol. 87, No. 3, pp. 305-335.

24. Ibid.

25. Ilana M. Horwitz, "Religion and Academic Achievement: A Research Review Spanning Secondary School and Higher Education," *Review of Religious Research*, Oct. 2020, Vol. 63, pp. 107-154.

26. Ilana M. Horwitz, Benjamin W. Domingue, and Kathleen Mullan Harris, "Not a Family Matter: The Effects of Religiosity on Academic Outcomes Based on Evidence from Siblings," *Social Science Research*, May-July 2020, 102426.

27. "Effects of Religious Practice on Education," Marripedia, Marriage and Religion Research Institute, http://marripedia.org/effects_of_religious_practice_on_education.

28. W. Bradford Wilcox, Wendy Wang, and Ian Rowe, "Less Poverty, Less Prison, More College: What Two Parents Mean For Black and White Children," Institute for Family Studies, ifstudies.org, June 17, 2021.

29. William De Soto, Hassan Tajalli, Nathan Pino, and Chad L. Smith, "The Effect of College Students' Religious Involvement on Their Academic Ethic," *Religion & Education*, Feb. 2018, Vol. 45, No. 2, pp. 190-207.

30. Shannon Gwin, Paul Branscum, Laurette Taylor, Marshall Cheney, Sarah B Maness, Melissa Frey, and Ying Zhang, "Associations Between Depressive Symptoms and Religiosity in Young Adults," *Journal of Religion and Health*, Dec. 2020, Vol. 59, Issue 6, pp. 3193-3210.

31. "National College Heath Assessment—Reference Group Executive Summary," American College Health Association, Spring 2019 edition and Fall 2011 edition, https://www.acha.org/ACHA/Resources/Survey_Data/NCHA/NCHA/Data/Publications_and_Reports.aspx?hkey=42461a35-897f-4664-bde7-f2410d487ca5.

32. "Depression & College Students," Affordable Colleges Online, April 19, 2021, https://www.affordablecollegesonline.org/college-resource-center/college-student-depression/.

33. Ibid.

34. Quoted in Quinten K. Lynn, "Sacred Sport: A Study of Student Athletes' Sanctification of Sport," dissertation submitted to the Graduate College of Bowling Green State University in partial fulfillment of the requirements for the degree of doctor of philosophy, Dec. 2008.

35. Ibid.

36. Thomas Ashby Wills, Alison M. Yaeger, and James M. Sandy, "Buffering Effect of Religiosity for Adolescent Substance Use," *Psychology of Addictive Behaviors*, March 2003, Vol. 17, No. 1, 24-31.

37. Cited in Patrick F. Fagan, "Why Religion Matters: The Impact of Religious Practice on Social Stability," Backgrounder, The Heritage Foundation, Jan. 25, 1996.

38. Adam E. Barry, Danny Valdez, and Alex M. Russell, "Does Religiosity Delay Adolescent Alcohol Initiation? A Long-Term Analysis (2008-2015) of Nationally Representative Samples of 12th Graders," *Substance Use & Misuse*, Nov., 2019, Vol. 55, No. 3, pp. 503-511.

39. Jason Fletcher and Sanjeev Kumar, "Religion and Risky Health Behaviors Among U.S. Adolescents and Adults," *Journal of Economic Behavior & Organization*, Aug. 2014, Vol. 104, pp. 123-140.

40. Annette Mahoney, Daniel D. Flint, and James S. McGraw, "Spirituality, Religion, and Marital/Family Issues," in *Handbook of Spirituality, Religion, and Mental Health*, second edition, David H. Rosmarin and Harold G. Koenig (Eds.), Academic Press, an imprint of Elsevier, 2020.

41. Patrick F. Fagan, "Why Religion Matters: The Impact of Religious Practice on Social Stability," Backgrounder, The Heritage Foundation, Jan. 25, 1996.

Chapter 9: Church and Sex

1. Quoted in Thomas Lickona, "The Neglected Heart: The Emotional Dangers of Premature Sexual Involvement," Catholic Education Resource Center, https://www.catholiceducation.org/en/marriage-and-family/sexuality/the-neglected-heart-the-emotional-dangers-of-premature-sexual-involvement.html.

2. Kirk Johnson, Lauren Noyes, and Robert Rector, "Sexually Active Teenagers Are More Likely to Be Depressed and to Attempt Suicide," Center for Data Analysis Report #03-04, The Heritage Foundation, June 3, 2003.

3. With One Voice 2012; America's Adults and Teens Sound Off About Teen Pregnancy, The National Campaign to Prevent Teen and Unplanned Pregnancy.

4. Quoted in, Thomas Lickona, "The Neglected Heart: The Emotional Dangers of Premature Sexual Involvement," Catholic Education Resource Center.

5. Ibid.

6. Donald P. Orr, Mary Beiter, and Gary Ingersoll, "Premature Sexual Activity as an Indicator of Psychosocial Risk," *Pediatrics*, Feb. 1991, Vol. 87, No. 2, pp. 141-147.

7. Quoted in Thomas Lickona, "The Neglected Heart: The Emotional Dangers of Premature Sexual Involvement," Catholic Education Resource Center, https://www.catholiceducation.org/en/marriage-and-family/sexuality/the-neglected-heart-the-emotional-dangers-of-premature-sexual-involvement.html.

8. Ibid.

9. Miriam Grossman, *Unprotected: A Campus Psychiatrist Reveals How Political Correctness in Her Profession Endangers Every Student*, Sentinel, published by Penguin Group, New York, 2006, p. 85. (Originally published under the author name Anonymous, M.D.)

10. Priscilla K. Coleman, "Abortion and Mental Health: Quantitative Synthesis and Analysis of Research Published 1995-2009," *The British Journal of Psychiatry*, Sept. 2011, Vol. 199, Issue 3, pp. 180-186.

11. George Skelton, "Many in Survey Who Had Abortion Cite Guilt Feelings," *Los Angeles Times*, March 19, 1989.

12. "Consequences of the Sexual Revolution," Uplifting Education website, https://www.upliftingeducation.net/consequences-of-the-sexual-revolution, "Effects of STDs," Epigee website, http://www.epigee.org/effects-of-stds.html, Tracee Cornforth, "Common Risks With Sexually Transmitted Infections," Verywell Health website, https://www.verywellhealth.com/consequences-of-sexually-transmitted-diseases-3522616.

13. Peter S. Bearman and Hannah Brückner, "Promising the Future: Virginity Pledges and First Intercourse," *American Journal of Sociology*, Jan. 2001, Vol. 106, No. 4.

14. "Abortion's Effects on Physical and Mental Health," American Association of Christian Counselors website, Sept. 8, 2020, https://www.aacc.net/2020/09/08/abortions-effects-on-physical-and-mental-health/, "15 Dreadful Side Effects of Abortion for Women's Health," DrHealthBenefits.com, https://drhealthbenefits.com/pregnancy/pregnancy-complications/side-effects-of-abortion-for-womens-health.

15. Miriam Grossman, *Unprotected: A Campus Psychiatrist Reveals How Political Correctness in Her Profession Endangers Every Student*, Sentinel, published by Penguin Group, New York, 2006, p. 28, 30. (Originally published under the author name Anonymous, M.D.)

16. "The Invisible Effects of Sex Before Marriage?," Moral Revolution website, https://www.moralrevolution.com/blog/the-invisible-effects-of-sex-before-marriage/.

17. Dean M. Busby, Jason S. Carroll, and Brian J. Willoughby, "Compatibility or Restraint? The Effects of Sexual Timing on Marriage Relationships," *Journal of Family Psychology*, Dec. 2010, Vol. 24, No 6. 776-774.

18. Nicholas H. Wolfinger, "Does Sexual History Affect Marital Happiness?," Institute of Family Studies, Oct. 22, 2018.

19. Juliana E. French, Emma E. Altgelt, and Andrea L. Meltzer, "The Implications of Sociosexuality for Marital Satisfaction and Dissolution," *Psychological Science*, Sept., 2019.

20. Quoted in Thomas Lickona, "The Neglected Heart: The Emotional Dangers of Premature Sexual Involvement," Catholic Education Resource Center, https://www.catholiceducation.org/en/marriage-and-family/sexuality/the-neglected-heart-the-emotional-dangers-of-premature-sexual-involvement.html.

21. Kristin Moore, Anne Driscoll, and Laura Duberstein Lindberg, *A Statistical Portrait of Adolescent Sex, Contraception, and Childbearing*, March 1, 1998, National Campaign to Prevent Teen Pregnancy, Washington, D.C.

22. Ann M. Meier, "Adolescents' Transition to First Intercourse, Religiosity, and Attitudes About Sex," *Social Forces*, March 2003, Vol. 81, Issue 3.

23. Jennifer Manlove, Cassandra Logan, Kristin A. Moore, and Erum Ikramullah, "Pathways from Family Religiosity to Adolescent Sexual Activity and Contraceptive Use," *Perspectives on Sexual and Reproductive Health*, June 10, 2008, Vol. 40, No. 2.

24. Lynn Blinn-Pike, "Why Abstinent Adolescents Report They Have Not Had Sex: Understanding Sexually Resilient Youth," *Family Relations*, July 1999, Vol. 48, No. 3.

25. Peter S. Bearman and Hannah Brückner, "Promising the Future: Virginity Pledges and First Intercourse," *American Journal of Sociology*, Jan. 2001, Vol. 106, No. 4.
26. Hanna Rosin, "Even Evangelical Teens Do It: How Religious Beliefs Do, and Don't, Influence Sexual Behavior," *Slate*, May 30, 2007, https://slate.com/culture/2007/05/mark-regnerus-forbidden-fruit-sex-religion-in-the-lives-of-american-teenagers.html.
27. Jeremy E. Uecker, "Religion, Pledging, and the Premarital Sexual Behavior of Married Young Adults," *Journal of Marriage and Family*, Aug., 2008, Vol. 70, No. 3.
28. Jeremy E. Uecker, "Religion, Pledging, and the Premarital Sexual Behavior of Married Young Adults," *Journal of Marriage and Family*, Aug. 2008, Vol. 70, No. 3.
29. Charlotte Paul, Julie Fitzjohn, Jason Eberhart-Phillips, Peter Herbison, and Nigel Dickson, "Sexual Abstinence at Age 21 in New Zealand: The Importance of Religion," *Social Science & Medicine*, July 2000, Vol. 51, Issue 1.
30. Lynn Blinn-Pike, "Why Abstinent Adolescents Report They Have Not Had Sex: Understanding Sexually Resilient Youth," *Family Relations*, July 1999, Vol. 48, No. 3.
31. Sameera Ahmed, Wahiba Abu Ras, and Cynthia Arfken, "Prevalence of Risk Behaviors Among U.S. Muslim College Students," *Journal of Muslim Mental Health*, March 2014, Vol. 8, Issue 1.

Chapter 10: Staving Off Suicide

1. Noelle Garcia, "Getting Others to Heaven: Learning to be a Leader," audio recording, Lighthouse Catholic Media/Augustine Institute.
2. Patrick Hedlund, "City Worker Talks Suicidal Man Out of Jumping Off Washington Heights Bridge," DNAinfo.com, Oct. 8, 2010.
3. Miriam Grossman, *Unprotected: A Campus Psychiatrist Reveals How Political Correctness in Her Profession Endangers Every Student*, Sentinel, published by Penguin Group, New York, 2006, p. 40. (Originally published under the author name Anonymous, M.D.)
4. Steven Stack, "The Effect of Domestic/Religious Individualism on Suicide, 1954-1978," *Journal of Marriage and Family*, May 1985, Vol. 47, No. 2.
5. Francie Hart Broghammer, "Death by Loneliness," *RealClear Policy*, May 06, 2019, https://www.realclearpolicy.com/articles/2019/05/06/death_by_loneliness_111185.html.
6. Bob Unruh, "Dad Links Son's Suicide to 'The God Delusion'," *World Net Daily*, Nov. 20, 2008.
7. Thomas Bass, "Interview with Richard Dawkins," *Omni*, Jan. 1990.
8. Ken Hensley, "A Very Special Breed: How I Evangelize Those Who Doubt or Deny the Existence of God Part XII," The Coming Home Network International blog, Jan. 8, 2019, https://chnetwork.org/2019/01/08/a-very-special-breed-how-i-evangelize-those-who-doubt-or-deny-the-existence-of-god-part-xii/.
9. National Center for Health Statistics Data Brief No. 362, April 2020.
10. Gallup, https://news.gallup.com/poll/1690/religion.aspx.
11. "Increase in Suicide Mortality in the United States, 1999-2018" and "Suicide Mortality in the United States, 1999-2019," National Center for Health Statistics Data Brief nos. 362 and 398, April 2020 and Feb. 2021, National Center for Health Statistics.
12. Tyler VanderWeele, Shanshan Li, and Ichiro Kawachi, reply to letter to the edi-

tor concerning "Religious Service Attendance and Suicide Rates," *JAMA Psychiatry*, Feb. 2017, Vol. 74, Issue 2.

13. Tyler VanderWeele, e-mail communication with author, May 5, 2021.

14. Cited in Patrick F. Fagan, "Why Religion Matters Even More: The Impact of Religious Practice on Social Stability," Backgrounder, The Heritage Foundation, Dec. 18, 2006.

15. Paul A. Nisbet, Paul R. Duberstein, Yeates Conwell, and Larry Seidlitz, "The Effect of Participation in Religious Activities on Suicide Versus Natural Death in Adults 50 and Older," *The Journal of Nervous and Mental Disease*, Aug. 2000, Vol. 188, Issue 8.

16. Cited in Tyler J. VanderWeele, "Religion and Health: A Synthesis," In: Peteet, J.R. and Balboni, M.J. (Eds.), *Spirituality and Religion within the Culture of Medicine: From Evidence to Practice*, Oxford University Press, 2017.

17. Evan M. Kleiman and Richard T. Liu, "Prospective Prediction of Suicide in a Nationally Representative Sample: Religious Service Attendance as a Protective Factor," *The British Journal of Psychiatry*, 2014, Vol. 204, pp. 262-266.

18. Steven Stack, "The Effect of the Decline in Institutionalized Religion on Suicide, 1954-1978," *Journal for the Scientific Study of Religion*, Sept. 1983, Vol. 22, No. 3.

19. Kanita Dervic, Maria A. Oquendo, Michael F. Grunebaum, Steve Ellis, Ainsley K. Burke, and J. John Mann, "Religious Affiliation and Suicide Attempt," *American Journal of Psychiatry*, Dec. 2004, Vol. 161, No. 12.

20. Brett Pelham and Zsolt Nyiri, "In More Religious Countries, Lower Suicide Rates," Gallup news release, July 3, 2008.

21. Tyler J. VanderWeele, "Religion and Health: A Synthesis," In: Peteet, J.R. and Balboni, M.J. (Eds.), *Spirituality and Religion within the Culture of Medicine: From Evidence to Practice*, Oxford University Press, 2017.

22. Émile Durkheim, *Suicide: A Study in Sociology*, Routledge Classics, 2002, first published in 1897, p. 143, 168.

23. Sascha O. Becker and Ludger Woessmann, "Knocking on Heaven's Door? Protestantism and Suicide," CESifo Working Paper No. 3499, June 2011, www.cesifo.org.

24. Ibid.

25. Paul Tillich, *The Protestant Era*, University of Chicago Press, 1948. p. 227. Cited in Flávio Antônio da Silva Dontal, "The Value of the Sacrament of Penance and Reconciliation for Psychology," Master's thesis, Georgetown University, May 2016.

26. Flávio Antônio da Silva Dontal, "The Value of the Sacrament of Penance and Reconciliation for Psychology," Master's thesis, Georgetown University, May 2016.

27. Center for Applied Research in The Apostolate, Georgetown University, https://cara.georgetown.edu/reconciliation.pdf.

28. Tyler J. VanderWeele, Shanshan Li, Alexander C. Tsai, and Ichiro Kawachi, "Association Between Religious Service Attendance and Lower Suicide Rates Among US Women," *JAMA Psychiatry*, Aug. 2016, Vol. 73, Issue 8.

29. Sterling C. Hilton, Gilbert W. Fellingham, and Joseph L. Lyon, "Suicide Rates and Religious Commitment in Young Adult Males in Utah," *American Journal of Epidemiology*, March 2002, Vol. 155, Issue 5, pp. 413-419.

30. Rachel Woodlock, "What Religions Really Say About Suicide," *Catholic San Francisco*, July 12, 2018, https://catholic-sf.org/news/what-religions-really-say-about-suicide.

31. David Bukay, "The Religious Foundations of Suicide Bombings," *Middle East Quarterly*, Fall 2006, Vol. 13, No. 4; Michael Rubin, "Why So Many Suicide Bombers If Islam Prohibits Suicide?," American Enterprise Institute blog, Jan. 12, 2015.
32. Jayaram V., "About Suicides in Hinduism," Hinduwebsite.com.
33. "What is the Buddhist Perspective on Suicide?," One Life Five Precepts, https://ethics.buddhist.sg/; Sara Conover, "Ask A Buddhist: What Happens to Someone after Suicide?," Spokanefavs.com, Feb. 28, 2018.
34. Jie Zhang and Huilan Xu, "The Effects of Religion, Superstition, and Perceived Gender Inequality on the Degree of Suicide Intent: A Study of Serious Attempters in China," *OMEGA - Journal of Death and Dying*, 2007, Vol. 55, No. 3, pp. 185-197.
35. "How Do Hindus Worship?," Reference.com, Mar. 28, 2020, https://www.reference.com/world-view/hindus-worship-551ecf4561a795d5.
36. Lee-Peng Kok, "Race, Religion and Female Suicide Attempters in Singapore," *Social Psychiatry and Psychiatric Epidemiology*, Dec. 1988, Vol 23, pages 236-239.
37. Andrew Wu, Jing-Yu Wang, and Cun-Xian Jia, "Religion and Completed Suicide: a Meta-Analysis," *PLoS ONE*, June 2015, Vol. 10, Issue 6.

Chapter 11: Church Lifts Poor and Minorities

1. Mary Fairchild, "Read Short 'Popcorn' Testimonies of Transformed Lives," LearnReligions.com, Aug. 27, 2020, https://www.learnreligions.com/popcorn-testimonies-701459.
2. "Child Poverty Rate in the U.S. from 1990 to 2019," Statistica.com.
3. Byron R. Johnson, Ralph Brett, and Derek Webb, *Objective Hope: Assessing the Effectiveness of Faith-Based Organizations*, Center for Research on Religion and Urban Civil Society, University of Pennsylvania, 2002.
4. Allan F Abrahamse, Peter A Morrison, and Linda J Waite, "Beyond Stereotypes: Who Becomes a Single Teenage Mother," Rand Corporation, 1988.
5. Cited in Patrick F. Fagan, "Why Religion Matters: The Impact of Religious Practice on Social Stability," Backgrounder, The Heritage Foundation, Jan. 25, 1996.
6. W. Bradford Wilcox and Nicholas H. Wolfinger, "Then Comes Marriage? Religion, Race, and Marriage in Urban America," *Social Science Research*, June 2007, Vol. 36, No. 2.
7. Ibid.
8. Cited in Jonathan Gruber, "Religious Market Structure, Religious Participation, and Outcomes: Is Religion Good for You?," National Bureau of Economic Research working paper 11377, May 2005.
9. Christopher G. Ellison, Amy M. Burdette, and W. Bradford Wilcox, "The Couple that Prays Together: Race and Ethnicity, Religion, and Relationship Quality Among Working-Age Adults," *Journal of Marriage and Family*, Aug 2010, Vol. 72, No. 4, pp. 963-975.
10. W. Bradford Wilcox and Nicholas H. Wolfinger, "Then Comes Marriage? Religion, Race, and Marriage in Urban America," *Social Science Research*, June 2007, Vol. 36, No. 2.
11. Amy C. Butler, "Welfare, Premarital Childbearing, and the Role of Normative Climate: 1968-1994," *Journal of Marriage and Family*, May 2002, Vol. 64, No. 2.
12. Amy M. Burdette, Stacy Haynes, and Christopher G. Ellison, "Religion, Race/Ethnicity, and Barriers to Marriage Among Working-Age Adults," National Center for Family and Marriage Research – Bowling Green State University Working

Paper Series WP-10-11, Sept. 2010.

13. W. Bradford Wilcox and Nicholas H. Wolfinger, "Then Comes Marriage? Religion, Race, and Marriage in Urban America," *Social Science Research*, June 2007, Vol. 36, Issue 2.

14. Diana Mendley Rauner, *They Still Pick Me Up When I Fall: The Role of Caring in Youth Development and Community Life*, Columbia University Press, New York, 2000, p. 118.

15. Mark D. Regnerus and Glen H. Elder, Jr., "Staying on Track in School: Religious Influences in High- and Low-Risk Settings," *Journal for the Scientific Study of Religion*, Dec. 2003, Vol. 42, No. 4.

16. Elijah Anderson, *Code of the Street: Decency, Violence, and The Moral Life of The Inner City*, W. W. Norton, 1999, p. 60.

17. Mark D. Regnerus and Glen H. Elder, Jr., "Staying on Track in School: Religious Influences in High- and Low-Risk Settings," *Journal for the Scientific Study of Religion*, Dec. 2003, Vol. 42, No. 4.

18. Ivory Toldson and Kenneth Alonzo Anderson, "Editor's Comment: The Role of Religion in Promoting Academic Success for Black Students," *The Journal of Negro Education*, Summer 2010, Vol 79, No. 3.

19. "John Pridmore's Testimony: From Drug Gangs to Christ," *Parousia*, parousia-media.com, Oct. 2, 2018.

20. Richard B. Freeman and Harry J. Holzer, eds., *The Black Youth Employment Crisis*, National Bureau of Economic Research Project Report, University of Chicago Press, 1986, p. 13.

21. Naida M. Parson and James K. Mikawa, "Incarceration and Non-Incarceration of African American Men Raised in Black Christian Churches," *Journal of Psychology*, 1991, Vol. 125, Issue 2, pp. 163-173.

22. Byron R. Johnson, Ralph Brett, and Derek Webb, *Objective Hope: Assessing the Effectiveness of Faith-Based Organizations, Center for Research on Religion and Urban Civil Society*, University of Pennsylvania, 2002.

23. Byron R. Johnson and Marc B. Siegel, *The Great Escape: How Religion Alters the Delinquent Behavior of High-Risk Adolescents*, Baylor ISR Report, 2008. Baylor Institute for Studies in Religion.

24. "Parental Religious Devotion Protects Against Major Delinquency," National Study of Youth and Religion, youthandreligion.nd.edu.

25. Byron R. Johnson, Ralph Brett, and Derek Webb, *Objective Hope: Assessing the Effectiveness of Faith-Based Organizations*, Center for Research on Religion and Urban Civil Society, University of Pennsylvania, 2002.

26. Christopher G. Ellison and Kristin L. Anderson, "Religious Involvement and Domestic Violence Among U.S. Couples," *Journal for the Scientific Study of Religion*, June 2001. Vol. 40, No. 2.

27. Byron R. Johnson, Ralph Brett, and Derek Webb, *Objective Hope: Assessing the Effectiveness of Faith-Based Organizations*, Center for Research on Religion and Urban Civil Society, University of Pennsylvania, 2002.

Chapter 12: Not All Spirituality is Equal

1. Mia Dinoto, "My Testimony | How Jesus Saved Me From Anorexia, Anxiety & Depression," YouTube, Jan. 11, 2021, https://youtu.be/9Xtc5PyzCUA.

2. Andrew Newberg, "Mind and God: The New Science of Neurotheology," *Big Think*, May 6, 2021, https://bigthink.com/mind-brain/mind-god-new-science-neurotheology.

3. Tyler VanderWeele, telephone interview with author, March 1, 2021.

4. "Frequency of Religious Attendance: 'A Powerful Social Determinant of Health'," *Crossroads,* newsletter of the Center for Spirituality, Theology and Health, Duke University, Vol. 10, Issue 3, Sept. 2020.

5. Marc A. Musick, James S. House, and David R. Williams, "Attendance at Religious Services and Mortality in a National Sample," *Journal of Health and Social Behavior,* June 2004, Vol. 45, No. 2, pp. 198-213.

6. Marilyn Baetz, Rudy Bowen, Glenn Jones, and Tulay Koru-Sengul, "How Spiritual Values and Worship Attendance Relate to Psychiatric Disorders in the Canadian Population," *Canadian Journal of Psychiatry,* Sept. 2006, Vol. 51, No. 10, pp. 654-661.

7. Michael King, Louise Marston, Sally McManus, Terry Brugha, Howard Meltzer, and Paul Bebbington, "Religion, Spirituality and Mental Health: Results From a National Study of English Households," *The British Journal of Psychiatry,* 2013, Vol. 202, pp. 68-73.

8. Chaeyoon Lim and Robert D. Putnam, "Religion, Social Networks, and Life Satisfaction," *American Sociological Review,* Dec. 2010, Vol. 75, No. 6 pp. 914-933.

9. Ying Chen and Tyler J. VanderWeele, "Associations of Religious Upbringing With Subsequent Health and Well-Being From Adolescence to Young Adulthood: An Outcome-Wide Analysis," *American Journal of Epidemiology,* Sept. 2018, Vol. 187, No. 11.

10. Scott A. Desmond, "Secrets and Lies: Adolescent Religiosity and Concealing Information from Parents," *Religions,* Feb. 2019, Vol. 10, Issue 2, p. 132.

11. "1.2F Durkheim and Social Integration," Social Science LibreTexts, https://socialsci.libretexts.org/.

12. Marc A. Musick, James S. House, and David R. Williams, "Attendance at Religious Services and Mortality in a National Sample," *Journal of Health and Social Behavior,* June 2004, Vol. 45, No. 2, pp. 198-213.

13. Steven R. Hemler, "Why We Need the Church," video presentation, CMAX.TV, 2020.

14. Harold Koenig, telephone interview with author, March 16, 2021.

15. Michael E. McCullough and Brian L.B. Willoughby, "Religion, Self-Regulation, and Self-Control: Associations, Explanations, and Implications," *Psychological Bulletin,* 2009, Vol. 135, No. 1, pp. 69-93.

16. Gordon W. Allport, *The Person in Psychology: Selected Essays,* Beacon Press, Boston, 1968, p. 150, cited in Fagan, "Why Religion Matters: The Impact of Religious Practice on Social Stability"; Gordon W. Allport and J. Michael Ross, "Personal Religious Orientation and Prejudice," *Journal of Personality and Social Psychology,* 1967, Vol. 5, 432-443.

17. Harold G. Koenig, Linda K. George, and Bercedis L. Peterson, "Religiosity and Remission of Depression in Medically Ill Older Patients," *American Journal of Psychiatry,* April 1998, Vol. 155, No. 4.

18. Thomas E. Oxman, Daniel H. Freeman Jr., and Eric D. Manheimer, "Lack of Social Participation or Religious Strength and Comfort as Risk Factors for Death After Cardiac Surgery in the Elderly," *Psychosomatic Medicine,* Jan.-Feb. 1995, Vol. 57, Issue 1, pp. 5-15. Also: "Harold Koenig | Spirituality into Clinical Practice," YouTube video, Feb. 4, 2020, https://www.youtube.com/watch?v=hb0nEaeqAjU&t=1951s.

19. Patrick F. Fagan, "Why Religion Matters Even More: The Impact of Religious Practice on Social Stability," Backgrounder, The Heritage Foundation, Dec. 18, 2006.

Also: "Why Religion Matters: The Impact of Religious Practice on Social Stability,"
The Heritage Foundation, Jan. 25, 1996.
20. Gordon W. Allport and J. Michael Ross, "Personal Religious Orientation and
Prejudice," *Journal of Personality and Social Psychology*, 1967, Vol. 5, 432-443.
21. Patrick F. Fagan, "Why Religion Matters: The Impact of Religious Practice on
Social Stability," Backgrounder, The Heritage Foundation, Jan. 25, 1996.
22. Ibid.

Chapter 13: Supernatural Graces

1. Dale A. Matthews, M.D. with Connie Clark, *The Faith Factor: Proof of the Healing
Power of Prayer*, Viking; The Penguin Group, 1998, p. 80.
2. Brendan O'Regan and Caryle Hirschberg, "Spontaneous Remission: An Annotat-
ed Bibliography," Institute of Noetic Sciences, 1993.
3. John A. Astin, Elaine Harkness, and Edzard Ernst, "The Efficacy of "Distant Randomized Trials," *Annals of Internal Medicine*, June 2000, Vol. 132, No. 11.
4. Leanne Roberts, Irshad Ahmed, and Steve Hall, "Intercessory Prayer for the
Alleviation of Ill Health," *Cochrane Database of Systematic Reviews*, April 2009.
5. Jeff Levin, *Religion and Medicine: A History of the Encounter Between Humanity's
Two Greatest Institutions*, Oxford University Press, 2020, p. 88.
6. R. B. Byrd, "Positive Therapeutic Effects of Intercessory Prayer in a Coronary Care
Unit Population," *Southern Medical Journal*, July 1988, Vol. 81, No. 7, pp. 826-829.
7. Christopher G. Ellison and Jeffery S. Levin, "The Religion-Health Connection:
Evidence, Theory, and Future Directions," *Health Education & Behavior*, Dec. 1998,
Vol. 25, No. 6, pp. 700-720.
8. W.J. Matthews, J.M. Conti, and S.G. Sireci, "The Effects of Intercessory Prayer,
Positive Visualization, and Expectancy on the Well-Being of Kidney Dialysis Patients," *Alternative Therapies in Health and Medicine*, 2001, Vol. 7, Issue 5.
9. Karen T Lesniak, "The Effect of Intercessory Prayer on Wound Healing in Non-
human Primates," *Alternative Therapies in Health and Medicine*, Nov-Dec. 2006, Vol.
12, No. 6, pp. 42-8.
10. "Time's Arrow: Albert Einstein's Letters to Michele Besso," Christies.com,
Nov. 14, 2017, https://www.christies.com/features/Einstein-letters-to-Michele-Bes-
so-8422-1.aspx.
11. Leonard Leibovici, "Effects of Remote, Retroactive Intercessory Prayer On Outcomes in Patients With Bloodstream Infection: Randomised Controlled Trial," Dec.
2001, *The BMJ*, Dec. 2001, Vol. 323, Issue 7327, pp. 1450-1451.
12. Brian Olshansky and Larry Dossey, "Retroactive Prayer: A Preposterous Hypothesis?," *The BMJ*, Nov. 30, 2003, Vol. 327, Issue 7429, pp. 1465-1468.
13. Mitchell W. Krucoff, Suzanne W. Crater, Dianne Gallup, James C. Blankenship,
Michael Cuffe, Mimi Guarneri, Richard A. Krieger, Vib R. Kshettry, Kenneth Morris,
Mehmet Oz, Augusto Pichard, Michael H. Sketch Jr., Harold G. Koenig, Daniel Mark,
and Kerry L. Lee, "Music, Imagery, Touch, and Prayer as Adjuncts to Interventional
Cardiac Care: The Monitoring and Actualisation of Noetic Trainings MANTRA II
Randomised Study," *The Lancet*, July 2005, Vol. 366, Issue 9481, pp. 211-17.
14. Mitchell W. Krucoff, Suzanne W. Crater, Cindy L. Green, Arthur C. Maas, Jon E.
Seskevich, James D. Lane, Karen A. Loeffler, Kenneth Morris, Thomas M. Bashore,
and Harold G. Koenig, "Integrative Noetic Therapies as Adjuncts to Percutaneous
Intervention During Unstable Coronary Syndromes: Monitoring and Actualization

of Noetic Training (MANTRA) Feasibility Pilot," *American Heart Journal*, Nov. 2001.
15. "Can Prayer Assist Healing?," Is-There-a-God.com, Feb. 17, 2017, https://www.
is-there-a-god.info/life/ipresults/

Chapter 14: Caveats to Consider

1. Kenneth I. Pargament, Harold G. Koenig, Nalini Tarakeshwar, and June Hahn,
"Religious Struggle as a Predictor of Mortality Among Medically Ill Elderly Patients:
A 2-Year Longitudinal Study," *JAMA Internal Medicine*, 2001, Vol. 161, No. 15, 1881-
1885.
2. Lynda H. Powell, Leila Shahabi, and Carl E. Thoresen, "Religion and Spirituality: Linkages to Physical Health," *American Psychologist*, Jan. 2003.
3. Christina Rush, Kaitlyn Vagnini, and Amy Wachholtz, "Spirituality/Religion and
Pain," in *Handbook of Spirituality, Religion, and Mental Health*, second edition, David H.
Rosmarin and Harold G. Koenig (Eds.), Academic Press, an imprint of Elsevier, 2020.
4. Claudia Kalb, "Faith & Healing," *Newsweek*, Nov. 9, 2003, https://www.news-
week.com/faith-healing-133365.
5. Kenneth I. Pargament, Harold G. Koenig, Nalini Tarakeshwar, and June Hahn,
"Religious Struggle as a Predictor of Mortality Among Medically Ill Elderly Patients: A
2-Year Longitudinal Study," *JAMA Internal Medicine*, 2001, Vol. 161, No. 15, 1881-1885.
6. Bruno Paz Mosqueiro, Alexandre de Rezende Pinto, and Alexander Morei-
ra-Almeida, "Spirituality, Religion, and Mood Disorders," also: Jonathan S.
Abramowitz, and Jennifer L. Buchholz, "Spirituality/Religion and Obsessive-Com-
pulsive-Related Disorders," *Handbook of Spirituality, Religion, and Mental Health*,
second edition, David H. Rosmarin and Harold G. Koenig (Eds.), Elsevier Inc.,
2020; also: Harold G. Koenig, *Is Religion Good for Your Health? The Effects of Religion
on Physical and Mental Health*, The Haworth Pastoral Press, 1997, pp. 106-108.
7. Harold G. Koenig, *Is Religion Good for Your Health? The Effects of Religion on Physical and Mental Health*, The Haworth Pastoral Press, 1997, p. 111.
8. Simon Dein, "Religion, Spirituality, and Mental Health," *Psychiatric Times*, Jan.
10, 2010, Vol 27, No 1.
9. Lee Strobel, *The Case for Christ: A Journalist's Personal Investigation of the Evidence
for Jesus*, Zondervan, 1998.
10. Simon Dein, "Religion, Spirituality, and Mental Health," *Psychiatric Times*, Jan.
10, 2010, Vol 27, No 1.
11. Mary B. Short, Thomas E. Kasper, and Chad T. Wetterneck, "The Relationship
Between Religiosity and Internet Pornography Use," *Journal of Religion and Health*,
April 2015, Vol. 54, No. 2, pp. 571-583.
12. Annette Mahoney, Kenneth I. Pargament, Aaron Murray-Swank, and Nichole
Murray-Swank, "Religion and the Sanctification of Family Relationships," *Review of
Religious Research*, March 2003, Vol. 44, No. 3, 220-236.
13. Cited in Annette Mahoney, Kenneth I. Pargament, Aaron Murray-Swank, and
Nichole Murray-Swank, "Religion and the Sanctification of Family Relationships,"
Review of Religious Research, March 2003, Vol. 44, No. 3, 220-236.
14. Annette Mahoney, Kenneth I. Pargament, Aaron Murray-Swank, and Nichole
Murray-Swank, "Religion and the Sanctification of Family Relationships," *Review of
Religious Research*, March 2003, Vol. 44, No. 3, 220-236.
15. Roy H. Schoeman, *Salvation is From the Jews*, Ignatius Press, 2003, pp. 147-175
(Kindle edition).

Chapter 15: Religion and Your Doctor

1. "Spirituality and Health," John Templeton Foundation, http://capabilities.templeton.org/2004/spirit01A.html.
2. Harold G. Koenig, *Is Religion Good for Your Health? The Effects of Religion on Physical and Mental Health*, The Haworth Pastoral Press, 1997, pp. 5-6.
3. Ibid., p. 7.
4. Jeff Levin, *Religion and Medicine: A History of the Encounter Between Humanity's Two Greatest Institutions*, Oxford University Press, 2020, p. 93.
5. Harold Koenig, telephone interview with author, March 16, 2021. Also see his paper "Religion, Spirituality, and Health: The Research and Clinical Implications," *ISRN Psychiatry*, Dec. 2012, Article ID 278730.
6. Harold Koenig, telephone interview with author, March 16, 2021.
7. Abdu'l-Missagh Ghadirian, Medicine and Spirituality blog, http://www.medicineandspirituality.com/; David Lewellen, "Medical Schools Explore Spirituality," *Health Progress*, Nov.-Dec. 2016, chausa.org.
8. Simon Dein, "Religion, Spirituality, and Mental Health," *Psychiatric Times*, Jan 10, 2010, Vol. 27, No 1.
9. Harold G. Koenig, "Religion and Medicine II: Religion, Mental Health, and Related Behaviors," *International Journal of Psychiatry in Medicine*, 2001, Vol. 31, No. 1, 97-109.
10. Christopher G. Ellison and Jeffrey S. Levin, "The Religion-Health Connection: Evidence, Theory, and Future Directions," *Health Education & Behavior*, Dec. 1998, Vol. 25, No. 6, pp. 700-720.
11. Cited in Loyd S. Wright, Christopher J Frost, and Stephen J. Wisecarver, "Church Attendance, Meaningfulness of Religion, and Depressive Symptomatology Among Adolescents," *Journal of Youth and Adolescence*, Jan. 1993, Vol. 22, No. 5, 559-568.
12. Ibid.
13. Patrick F. Fagan, "Why Religion Matters: The Impact of Religious Practice on Social Stability," Backgrounder, The Heritage Foundation, Jan. 25, 1996.
14. Kanita Dervic, Maria A. Oquendo, Michael F. Grunebaum, Steve Ellis, Ainsley K. Burke, and J. John Mann, "Religious Affiliation and Suicide Attempt," *American Journal of Psychiatry*, Dec. 2004, Vol. 161, No. 12.
15. Simon Dein, "Religion, Spirituality, and Mental Health," *Psychiatric Times*, Jan. 10, 2010, Vol. 27, No 1.
16. Christopher G. Ellison and Jeffrey S. Levin, "The Religion-Health Connection: Evidence, Theory, and Future Directions," *Health Education & Behavior*, Dec. 1998, Vol. 25, No. 6, 700-720.
17. https://en.wikipedia.org/wiki/Albert_Ellis#cite_note-31.
18. See Harold Koenig, "Religion, Spirituality, and Health: The Research and Clinical Implications," *ISRN Psychiatry*, Dec. 2012, Article ID 278730.
19. Simon Dein, Christopher C. H. Cook, Andrew Powell, and Sarah Eagger, "Religion, Spirituality, and Mental Health," *The Psychiatrist*, 2010, Vol. 34, 63-64.
20. "Religiosity, Income, Health and Life Satisfaction," *Crossroads*, newsletter of the Center for Spirituality, Theology and Health, Duke University, Vol. 9, Issue 9, March 2020.
21. L. Rebecca Propst, Richard Ostrom, Philip Watkins, Terri Dean, and David Mashburn, "Comparative Efficacy of Religious and Nonreligious Cognitive-Behavioral Therapy for the Treatment of Clinical Depression in Religious Individuals," *Journal of Consulting and Clinical Psychology*, 1992, Vol. 60, No. 1, 94-103.

22. Philippe Huguelet, "Spirituality, Religion, and Psychotic Disorders," *Handbook of Spirituality, Religion, and Mental Health,* second edition, David H. Rosmarin and Harold G. Koenig (Eds.), Elsevier Inc., 2020.

23. Tyler J. VanderWeele, Shanshan Li, Alexander C. Tsai, and Ichiro Kawachi, "Association Between Religious Service Attendance and Lower Suicide Rates Among US Women, *JAMA Psychiatry,* Aug. 2016, Vol. 73, Issue 8.

24. Ibid.

25. Andrew Newberg, "The Spiritual Brain: Science and Religious Experience," The Great Courses series, lecture 10, July 2013.

26. Harold Koenig, "Maintaining Health and Well-Being by Putting Faith into Action During the COVID-19 Pandemic," *Journal of Religion and Health,* May 2020, Vol. 59, pp. 2205-2214.

27. Claudia Kalb, "Faith & Healing," *Newsweek,* Nov. 9, 2003, https://www.newsweek.com/faith-healing-133365.

28. Lynda H. Powell, Leila Shahabi, and Carl E. Thoresen, "Religion and Spirituality: Linkages to Physical Health," *American Psychologist,* Jan. 2003.

29. Claudia Kalb, "The Critic: 'Religion Is A Private Matter'," *Newsweek,* Nov. 9, 2003, http://www.newsweek.com/faith-healing-133365.

30. Tyler J. VanderWeele, "Religion and Health: A Synthesis," In: Peteet, J.R. and Balboni, M.J. (Eds.), *Spirituality and Religion within the Culture of Medicine: From Evidence to Practice,* Oxford University Press, 2017.

31. Tyler J. VanderWeele, "Religion and Health: A Synthesis," In: Peteet, J.R. and Balboni, M.J. (Eds.), *Spirituality and Religion within the Culture of Medicine: From Evidence to Practice,* Oxford University Press, 2017.

32. "Spirituality and Health," John Templeton Foundation, http://capabilities.templeton.org/2004/spirit01A.html.

33. Claudia Kalb, "The Advocate: 'Patients Want To Be Talked To'," *Newsweek,* Nov. 9, 2003, https://www.newsweek.com/advocate-patients-want-be-talked-133401.

34. Claudia Kalb, "Faith & Healing," *Newsweek,* Nov. 9, 2003, https://www.newsweek.com/faith-healing-133365.

35. Harold Koenig, telephone interview with author, March 16, 2021.

Chapter 16: Healthy Self and Citizenry

1. Patrick F. Fagan, "Why Religion Matters: The Impact of Religious Practice on Social Stability," Backgrounder, The Heritage Foundation, Jan. 25, 1996.

2. "Most Americans Practice Charitable Giving, Volunteerism," Gallup, Dec. 13, 2013, https://news.gallup.com/poll/166250/americans-practice-charitable-giving-volunteerism.aspx.

3. http://www.marripedia.org/_media/charity_and_volunteering.png.

4. Robert D. Putnam and David E. Campbell, *American Grace: How Religion Divides and Unites Us,* Simon & Schuster, 2012, p. 451, 461.

5. S. Philip Morgan, "A Research Note on Religion and Morality: Are Religious People Nice People?," *Social Forces,* March 1983, Vol. 61, No. 3.

6. Robert D. Putnam and David E. Campbell, *American Grace: How Religion Divides and Unites Us,* Simon & Schuster, 2012, p. 471, 468.

7. David E. Campbell, e-mail communication with author, Nov. 20, 2020.

8. Lee Strobel, *A Journalist's Personal Investigation of the Evidence for Jesus,* documentary, La Mirada films, 2007. And: Lee Strobel, *The Case for Christ: A Journalist's Personal Investigation of the Evidence for Jesus*, Zondervan, 1998, pp. 14, 273.

9. Cited in Michael E. McCullough and Brian L.B. Willoughby, "Religion, Self-Regulation, and Self-Control: Associations, Explanations, and Implications," *Psychological Bulletin*, 2009, Vol. 135, No. 1, 69-93.

10. Michael E. McCullough and Brian L.B. Willoughby, "Religion, Self-Regulation, and Self-Control: Associations, Explanations, and Implications," *Psychological Bulletin*, 2009, Vol. 135, No. 1, 69-93.

11. Ibid.

12. Azim Shariff and Ara Norenzayan, "God Is Watching You: Priming God Concepts Increases Prosocial Behavior in an Anonymous Economic Game," *Psychological Science*, 2007, Vol 18, No. 9.

13. Quoted in Owen Chadwick, *The Secularization of the European Mind in the Nineteenth Century*, Cambridge University Press, 1975, p. 10.

14. Bruce Sheiman, *An Atheist Defends Religion: Why Humanity is Better Off with Religion than without It*, Alpha Books, a division of Penguin, 2009, p. 70, p. vii.

15. "Atheist Alain de Botton Challenges Hitchens' Assertion that 'Religion Poisons Everything'," *National Post*, March 10, 2012, https://nationalpost.com/holy-post/atheist-alain-de-botton-challenges-hitchens-assertion-that-religion-poisons-everything.

16. Michael S. Rose, *Ugly As Sin: Why They Changed Our Churches from Sacred Places to Meeting Spaces, and How We Can Change Them Back Again*, Sophia Institute Press, 2001.

17. Michael Fitzgerald, "Satan, the Great Motivator: The Curious Economic Effects of Religion," *The Boston Globe*, Nov. 15, 2009, http://www.boston.com/bostonglobe/ideas/articles/2009/11/15/the_curious_economic_effects_of_religion/?page=full.

18. Robert J. Barro and Rachel McCleary, "Religion and Economic Growth," *American Sociological Review*, June 2003, Vol. 68, No. 464.

19. Ibid.

20. Michael Fitzgerald, "Satan, the Great Motivator: The Curious Economic Effects of Religion," *The Boston Globe*, Nov. 15, 2009, http://www.boston.com/bostonglobe/ideas/articles/2009/11/15/the_curious_economic_effects_of_religion/?page=full.

21. Patrick F. Fagan, "Why Religion Matters: The Impact of Religious Practice on Social Stability," Backgrounder, The Heritage Foundation, Jan. 25, 1996.

22. Michael Fitzgerald, "Satan, the Great Motivator: The Curious Economic Effects of Religion," *The Boston Globe*, November 15, 2009.

23. Bruce Sheiman, *An Atheist Defends Religion: Why Humanity is Better Off with Religion than without It*, Alpha Books, a division of Penguin, 2009, p. 24.

24. James Q. Wilson, "In the Pew Instead of Prison," *The Wall Street Journal*, May 9, 2011.

25. Patrick F. Fagan, "Why Religion Matters Even More: The Impact of Religious Practice on Social Stability," Backgrounder, The Heritage Foundation, Dec. 18, 2006.

Chapter 17: Reasons to Believe

1. Tyler VanderWeele, Shanshan Li, and Ichiro Kawachi, reply to letter to the editor concerning "Religious Service Attendance and Suicide Rates," *JAMA Psychiatry*, Feb. 2017, Vol. 74, Issue 2. Also: Tyler VanderWeele, e-mail communication with author, May 5, 2021.

2. Ralph Lewis, "Profoundly Challenging Questions to Ask an Atheist," *Psychology Today*, Jan. 12, 2019.

3. Robert Jastrow, *God and the Astronomers*, second edition, 1992, W.W. Norton & Co., p. 14.

4. Robert Jastrow, *God and the Astronomers*, 1978, W.W. Norton & Co., p. 116.

5. Robert Jastrow, "A Scientist Caught Between Two Faiths," interview with Bill Durbin, *Christianity Today*, Aug. 6, 1982, p. 15, 18.

6. Stephen Hawking, *A Brief History of Time*, Bantam Dell Publishing Group, 1988.

7. Jay W. Richards, "List of Fine-Tuning Parameters," Jan. 14, 2015, Discovery Institute, https://www.discovery.org/a/fine-tuning-parameters/.

8. Geraint F. Lewis and Luke A. Barnes, *A Fortunate Universe: Life in a Finely Tuned Cosmos*, Author's Republic, 2016.

9. "Fine Tuning," interview of John Polkinghorne, YouTube, https://www.youtube.com/watch?v=ncsuh_5l6Hw.

10. Fred Hoyle, Intelligent Universe: A New View of Creation and Evolution, Holt Rinehart & Winston, 1983.

11. Michael Behe, *Darwin's Black Box: The Biochemical Challenge to Evolution*, Free Press, 1996; Also: Michael Behe, "Recognizing Design by a 'Purposeful Arrangement of Parts'," *Evolution News*, June 10, 2021, https://evolutionnews.org/2021/06/recognizing-design-by-a-purposeful-arrangement-of-parts/.

12. Douglas Axe, *Undeniable: How Biology Confirms Our Intuition That Life Is Designed*, HarperCollins, 2017, Chapter 2. Also: Douglas Axe, e-mail communication with author, April 11, 2021.

13. Francis Crick, *Life Itself: Its Origin and Nature*, New York: Simon & Schuster, 1981, p. 88.

14. Johnjoe McFadden and Jim Al-Khalili, *Life on the Edge: The Coming of Age of Quantum Biology*, Crown, 2016, p. 279-280.

15. Keith Ward, *Why There Is Almost Certainly a God*, Audible.com audio book. Also: "Religion and the Quantum World," Vimeo video, Gresham College lecture, March 9, 2005, https://vimeo.com/40154090.

16. Lee Strobel, *The Case for Christ: A Journalist's Personal Investigation of the Evidence for Jesus*, Zondervan, 1998, p. 249.

17. "What Were Christians Called Before St. Ignatius of Antioch Referred to Them as Catholics?," *Catholic Answers*, https://www.catholic.com/qa/what-were-christians-called-before-st-ignatius-of-antioch-referred-to-them-as-catholics.

18. Stephen Beale, "Just How Many Protestant Denominations Are There?," *National Catholic Register*, Oct. 31, 2017, https://www.ncregister.com/blog/just-how-many-protestant-denominations-are-there.

19. Michael E. Gaitley, *33 Days to Morning Glory*, Marian Press, 2015, p. 21.

20. C.G. Jung, *Critique of Psychoanalysis*, Princeton University Press, 1976, p. 110.

21. Cited in Flávio Antônio da Silva Dontal, "The Value of the Sacrament of Penance and Reconciliation for Psychology," Master's thesis, Georgetown University, May 2016.

22. Aaron Murray-Swank, "The Healing Practice of Confession," *Spirituality & Health*, Jan. 28, 2012, https://www.spiritualityhealth.com/articles/2012/01/28/healing-practice-confession.

23. "Finding Jesus' Touch Through Eucharistic Adoration," *The Catholic Register*, Dec. 3, 2007.

24. Thomas à Kempis, *The Imitation of Christ*, (originally composed 1418-1427), Hendrickson Publishers, 2004, p. 3.

Index

A

Abiders vs. Avoiders 125-126
abortion 91, 141-142, 199, 214
academic achievement 121-139
accountability partners 94
active goal pursuit 89
Add Health. *See* National Longitudinal Study of Adolescent Health
adolescents. *See* teenagers
African Americans 23, 36-37, 132, 148, 166
   religion-marriage paradox 166
agnosticism 64, 74, 80, 129, 203, 230
agreeableness 220
à Kempis, Thomas 246
Alabama and Mississippi 55
alcohol abuse 1-3, 7-8, 15, 17, 28, 76-79, 85, 92, 93, 96, 104, 111, 116, 122-123, 129, 131-
   132, 135, 138, 139-141, 148, 154, 161, 164, 168, 178, 213, 216
Alcoholics Anonymous 76
Aleaya's story. *See* personal stories
Al-Khalili, Jim 234
Allport, Gordon 183, 184
Al Shohaib, Saad Saleh 69
altruism 221, 222. *See also* volunteerism, charitable giving, good neighborliness,
   agreeableness
Alzheimer's disease 6, 36
American Grace: How Religion Divides and Unites Us 47, 217
American Journal of Psychiatry 2, 207
American Psychologist 50
American Sociological Review 2, 113
Anastasi, Matthew 71
An Atheist Defends Religion 222
Anderson, Elijah 165
Anderson, Kenneth Alonzo 170
Anderson, Kristin 173
anger 5, 38, 40-42, 45, 69, 71, 105, 113, 136, 162, 197, 202, 216
anterior cingulate cortex 61
anxiety 6, 25, 27, 33, 39, 41-43, 46, 61, 64, 68, 71, 72, 119, 135, 136, 141, 159, 175-177,
   183, 185, 197, 200, 213, 226, 246
apologetics 242, 245
art and architecture 223
assisted suicide 91
Astin, John 190
atheism 1-2, 9, 14, 15, 46, 58, 61, 64, 74, 76, 80-81, 83, 84, 119, 129, 152, 155, 198, 203,
   206, 208, 213, 219, 220, 222, 229, 230, 232, 234, 247
   church attendance and kids 129
athletes 89, 137, 138
Atkins, David 101
attention deficit hyperactivity disorder 89
autoimmune diseases 40
Axe, Douglas 233
Axinn, William 110-111, 113-114

B

Baetz, Marilyn 177
Bahr, Howard 98
Barro, Robert 224
Bartkowski, John 122
Baylor University 13, 27, 36, 172
Beach, Steven 105
Bearman, Peter 146
Beatitudes, The 215, 248
Beck, Aaron T. 73
Becker, Sascha 158
Benor, Daniel 190
Bering, Jesse 81
Bible, The 9, 16, 17, 22, 33, 38, 40, 55, 58, 68, 77, 94, 103, 104, 108, 113, 115, 118, 121, 131, 151, 157, 160, 175, 176, 180, 189, 205, 210, 215, 216, 219, 220, 224, 226, 236, 237, 239-241, 245, 248
  interpretation of 157, 240-241
Big Bang 231-232
Big Five dimensions of personality 220
binge drinking 7, 76. *See also* alcohol abuse
biology, cell. *See* intentional design in nature
Biswas-Diener, Robert 51
Blacks. *See* African Americans
Blessed Virgin Mary. *See* Mary, Blessed Virgin
Blinn-Pike, Lynn 145, 149
blood pressure 2, 26, 27, 28, 29, 30, 31, 35, 38, 41, 42, 71, 181, 185. *See also* cardiovascular
body mass index 29, 123
boundaries. *See* temptation resistance
Bowling Green State University 13, 107, 117, 137, 197, 200
Boyle, Patricia 36
brain 37, 59, 61, 65, 72, 85, 204
Brigham Young University 98, 143, 161
British Journal of Psychiatry, The 141
BMJ, The (British Medical Journal) 2, 192
Broghammer, Francie Hart 152
Bruce, Marino 27
Brückner, Hannah 146
Buddhism 29, 48, 72, 82, 150, 162, 190, 194-195, 224
Burdette, Amy 166
Busby, Dean 143
Byrd, Randolph 190

C

cafeteria Christians 102-103
Cairns-Smith, Graham 234
Call, Vaughn 98
Campbell, David 47, 217-219
cancer 1, 4, 6, 15, 20, 29, 30-31, 38, 41, 53, 142, 204
cardiovascular 6, 20, 26, 27, 29-31, 38, 39, 41-42, 48, 71, 105, 181, 185, 205, 228

kibbutzim, religious vs. secular 21-22, 225
Kilgore, Jessie 58, 152
Kim, Eric 48, 177
kindness. *See* good neighborliness
King, Valarie 115
Kleinman, Evan 154
Koenig, Harold G. 13, 17-18, 20, 28, 40, 53, 59, 62-63, 65, 69, 70-71, 77, 123, 154, 180, 183, 197, 204-206, 210, 212
Konrath, Sara 48
Koran. *See* Islam
Krause, Neal 37, 43, 44, 50
Krucoff, Mitchell 194

L

Lambert, Nathaniel 43, 63
Lancet, The 2, 209
Larson, David B. 18, 26-27, 206
Laurin, Kristin 85, 86
Lee, Kristen Schultz 129
Leibovici, Leonard 193
Levin, Jeff 13, 36, 39, 191, 205, 207, 208
Lewis, C.S. 11, 57
Lewis, Ralph 229
Lickona, Thomas 141
Lieberman, Louis 76
life expectancy 1, 8, 10, 12, 15, 16, 21-25, 27-30, 32, 48, 50, 64, 96, 177, 206
Life on the Edge: The Coming of Age of Quantum Biology 234
Lim, Chaeyoon 33, 52, 178
Lipitor 26, 211
Li, Shanshan 153
Liu, Richard 154
longevity. *See* life expectancy
Longevity Project, The 24, 25
longitudinal vs. cross-sectional studies 12
Lourdes, France. *See* Mary, Blessed Virgin, Lourdes miracles
Loury, Linda 130
low-income populations. *See* poor and disadvantaged
lukewarm religiosity 5, 14, 15, 29, 33, 34, 50, 74, 97-98, 101, 161, 176, 190
    compared with nonreligiosity 5, 34, 74, 98, 100, 160, 219
Luskin, Fred 41

M

Magis Center for Reason and Faith 56
Mahoney, Annette 13, 107, 117-201
Manhart, Michael 102
Manheimer, Eric 34
Manlove, Jennifer 145
Marbas, Laurie 18, 59
marriage 8, 3, 32, 75, 95, 95-111, 96-99, 101-111, 115, 117-119, 142-143, 146, 147-148, 165-167, 199-201, 242
    and health 95-96

About the Author

Patrick D. Chisholm is a former columnist for *The Christian Science Monitor* whose articles also have appeared in *The Washington Post, The Wall Street Journal, USA Today, Baltimore Sun, San Francisco Chronicle,* and other publications. He holds a B.A. in history and M.A. in international economics, and is a senior fellow with the Catholic Apologetics Institute of North America and board member of the Fatima Outreach Foundation. Perusing academic studies on the health benefits of religion prompted him years ago to become more active in matters of church and faith. Married with two boys, he lives in Chantilly, Virginia.

www.ingramcontent.com/pod-product-compliance
Lightning Source LLC
Chambersburg PA
CBHW060311030426
42336CB00011B/999